DIRT IS GOOD

DIRT IS GOOD

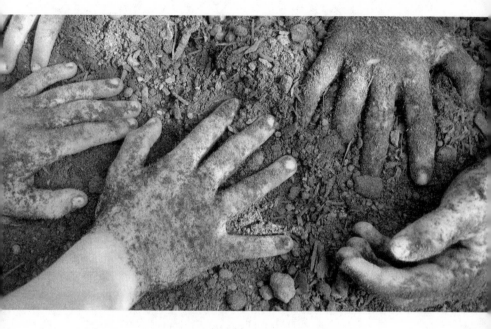

The Advantage of Germs for
Your Child's Developing Immune System

Jack Gilbert, Ph.D., and Rob Knight, Ph.D.

with Sandra Blakeslee

St. Martin's Press ⚲ New York

DIRT IS GOOD. Copyright © 2017 by Jack Anthony Gilbert, Rob Knight, and Sandra Blakeslee. All rights reserved. Printed in the United States of America. For information, address St. Martin's Press, 175 Fifth Avenue, New York, N.Y. 10010.

www.stmartins.com

Designed by Patrice Sheridan

Title page photograph: Varina C/Shutterstock.com

The Library of Congress Cataloging-in-Publication Data is available upon request

ISBN 978-1-250-13260-4 (hardcover)
ISBN 978-1-250-13262-8 (ebook)

Our books may be purchased in bulk for promotional, educational, or business use. Please contact the Macmillan Corporate and Premium Sales Department at 1-800-221-7945, extension 5442, or by e-mail at MacmillanSpecialMarkets@macmillan.com.

First Edition: June 2017

10 9 8 7 6 5 4 3 2 1

For our children

Contents

13. Conditions   190

14. Tests   213

DIRT IS GOOD

Introduction

"Is it okay for my kid to eat dirt?"

That's just one of the many questions we're bombarded with every day from parents all over the world who are worried about their children's health and confused about what they're reading on the Internet.

Why are they asking us?

Because we're two of the scientists leading the investigation of the human microbiome. That's often misunderstood as meaning "germs," but it's really the community of friendly microbes that populate the human body, as well as a few that, in the wrong context, aren't so good. This diverse multitude of tiny, invisible creatures helps us out in all kinds of ways, such as digesting food, making vitamins, protecting us from diseases, sculpting our organs, tuning our immune systems, and even shaping our behavior.

The notion that most bacteria, or germs, are intrinsically bad—and must be killed by any means possible—is widespread. But it's wrong, dangerously wrong. New methods of studying the microbial world reveal that most of the bacteria we encounter on a daily basis, and those that reside in and on our bodies, are not just friendly but even essential for keeping us alive. We exterminate them at our peril. In our zeal to vanquish all those classical plagues, we have inadvertently unleashed a Pandora's box of modern plagues—the array of slow-killing, miserable, chronic health problems that have become prevalent across the modern world: obesity, asthma, allergies, diabetes, celiac disease, irritable bowel syndrome, multiple sclerosis, rheumatoid arthritis, and many others.

The science of the microbiome is leading to fascinating discoveries, and in just the last few years it has gone from a wonkish subfield of biomedical research to a topic of intense public interest. You'll find it lionized in magazine and newspaper articles, TED talks (including ours), documentaries, radio and television talk shows, podcasts. And of course, it seems ubiquitous on the Internet, where it is inducing an enormous amount of hype and misinformation—and adding to the confusion and anxiety of parents who want to do the best for their young children.

Because of our expertise, we find ourselves being asked for our advice from all sorts of people in all sorts of situations.

After hearing a talk on the role of family dogs and a healthy microbiome, an audiovisual technician approaches the lectern. A bit nervously, he says, "My son loves our local playground, especially the sandbox and the jungle gym. He wants to go there every day. But the place looks filthy to me. I mean, gum wrappers, dog poop, pigeons everywhere. Should I worry about him catching a disease?"

After engaging in a short conversation about work, a balding taxi driver turns his head around and shoots a pained expression. "Oh my god, maybe you can help me. My son has diabetes. He's extremely overweight and he's only three. My wife and I don't know what to do."

A janitor at work stops us in the hall with a concerned look. "We're supposed to use antibacterial products on everything we clean, but is that a good idea? I work in two elementary schools and I have a five-year-old at home."

The questions pop up even when we're not being recognized for our expertise. In the Whole Foods supplements aisle a woman scrutinizing shelves of probiotics turns to ask, of anyone, "Do you have a clue as to which of these brands really work? My little girl has diarrhea. She's not getting better. I'm frantic!"

We can relate. In raising our own children, we have dealt with numerous frightening episodes where their health was challenged and we didn't know what to do, starting with birth itself. Each of our firstborns experienced rather terrifying (or at least we thought so at the time) events in the delivery room.

Jack's son, Dylan, was born in his own meconium, the dark greenish excrement produced by newborns. Because he had pooped in the birth canal, he was immediately given antibiotics and was kept in the hospital overnight for observation. This was done as a precaution against the possibility he had inhaled some of it, which in his new lungs could have caused a nasty infection. Dylan had multiple bouts of diarrhea by the time he was six months old and later suffered several flares of a yeast infection, or thrush, all over his body. This rash has raised white patches on a scarlet background. He had ear infections and developed a cry that always sounded like a bark or a cough. At age six, he was diagnosed with high-functioning autism, now increasingly linked to the microbiome.

When Rob's unborn daughter went into distress after a prolonged labor, the anxious parents reluctantly consented to a cesarean section. But they were not about to give up entirely on a vaginal delivery, which Rob's research strongly suggests confers benefits on newborns. An hour later, after the hospital staff had left them in their room alone, Rob pulled out some cotton swabs. Using these, he collected vaginal fluids from his partner Amanda and transferred them to his daughter's mouth, nose, ears, face, skin, and perineum. He inoculated her with her microbial birthright, which had been denied by the C-section. He did this because he had knowledge of the best available scientific evidence about what would be good for his newborn; he had even participated in that discovery.

Our goal in this book is to present you, too, with the best scientific advice available about the microbiome and your children's health and development. What procedures, drugs, foods, environmental exposures, and everyday practices can help or harm your children early in life? What can you do to protect their health and development? What works and what doesn't? How will you know if your child is heading in the right or wrong direction? What is being hyped and whom can you trust?

Not being medical doctors, we can't give medical advice. But as scientists who together have been involved in generating a substantial amount of the data that underlie the research that is now relied upon by physicians and other medical clinicians throughout the world, we can offer evidence-based answers to your questions and reliable ways to think about microbes and health. We answer these questions, where possible, with information about clinical trials performed in humans. However, often it's not possible or ethical to do the definitive experiment in humans, and in those cases we rely on a combination of observational studies (looking at differences between groups of people) and experiments in animals or in test-tube settings. Often, an observation in people (for example, that lean and obese people have different microbes) leads to detailed experiments (say, that mice given a particular microbe isolated from lean people will slim down itself). In general, this translation from bench to bedside allows us to know a lot more in terms of biological mechanisms than would be possible if we looked only at human studies. However, it's important to remember that the translation isn't always perfect, and the further you move away from a human study the less likely the results are to apply.

After a brief explanation of microbes and the human microbiome, we've organized this book to follow your child from pregnancy through birth and infancy, and then the toddler and preschool years. We pay special attention to medical conditions, assessments, and interventions that cut across those ages. Within each section, we answer the questions we are most commonly asked. You'll find that answers often lead right into the very next question you were about to ask, as well as its answer. We've tried our best to turn this book into a conversation, as if we were in the room with you.

Like it or not, the microbiome has permanently joined the long list of parental worries.

1

The Microbiome

Earth formed about 4.5 billion years ago when a disc-shaped cloud of dust and gas collapsed into a primordial sphere. It was lifeless and molten and reeked of lethal gases. When it finally cooled, a newly solid crust allowed liquid water (via special delivery from comets) to collect on the surface.

A billion years later, this hellish planet had been transformed. It was now slathered with free-living, single-cell organisms called prokaryotes and archaea. They amassed themselves into shallow microbial mats at the bottom of the ocean and on the sides of towering volcanoes. In fact, these original inhabitants survive to this day in the coldest and hottest regions of land and sea. And they can feed on just about anything, including ammonia, hydrogen, sulfur, and iron.

One of the great mysteries of biology is, how did all this life arise? How did nonliving chemicals manage to invent cell membranes and self-replication, to feed and repair themselves? Scientists used to think that a "primordial soup" was struck by lighting and suddenly organic life sparked into being—a la *Frankenstein*.

Current theories are only a little more prosaic. More recent evidence, based on a genetic analysis of known microbes, traces life's origins to deep-sea hydrothermal vents that spew out boiling gases.[1] In other words, the first cell we can know about by analyzing modern genes fed on hydrogen gas in a hot, pitch-dark, iron-rich, sulfurous environment. It had figured out how to obtain energy to live.

For millions of years, microbial mats pretty much ran things. Gradually, through countless real-life experiments driven by evolutionary forces, some of the microbes developed the ability to use the energy in sunlight to turn carbon dioxide and water into food. This process, known as photosynthesis, released massive amounts of oxygen. The air you breathe was made by those microbes. It still is.

We mention this background to help you get your head around a fact that is difficult to grasp: we humans live on a planet that is run by and for invisible microbes. For 3 billion years, they were its sole owners. They created our biosphere, maintaining global cycles involving carbon, nitrogen, sulfur, phosphorus, and other nutrients. They made all the soil. Last but not least, they set the conditions for the evolution of multicellular life, meaning plants and animals, including us.

The number of bacteria on Earth is estimated to be a nonillion: 10^{30} (10 to the 30th power, i.e., 10 followed by 30 zeros). That's more than the number of stars in our galaxy. The number of viruses is at least two orders of magnitude greater. According to a new estimate, there are about 1 trillion species of microbes on Earth and 99.999 percent of them have yet to be discovered.[2] If we lined them all up end to end, the "bug chain" would stretch to the Sun and back 200 trillion times.

That means all of microbiology is built on less than 1 percent of microbial life. We have only sequenced fifty thousand of their genomes for our databases. The rest are mysterious. We can't grow them in our labs. They have no names. Their functions are not known. We are surrounded by microbial dark matter.

Nevertheless, we have some pretty good ideas for how life operates and how simple rules give rise to complexity. All of biology is based on principles of evolution, competition, and cooperation. And microbes are masters at cooperation. The waste product of one microbe helps feed its neighbor. They care where they are and who is with them. And they share genetic information, passing it not only to their progeny but to their neighbors as well—even across species.

As for competition, the microbial world is a stage for endless war. Bugs that eat the same foods struggle to find ways to outwit their neighbors. As sworn enemies, bacteria and viruses have been duking it out for billions of years and, in so doing, have invented just about every chemical reaction, every defensive and offensive strategy imaginable, every survival trick in the book of life.

Organisms that we call microbes are grouped into three domains: Bacteria, Archaea, and Eukaryota. These domains are radically different from one another— far more different genetically than humans are from a squid or even a pine tree.

Microbes in the first domain, Bacteria, are what most of us think of when we talk about bugs or germs. They are single-cell organisms lacking a nucleus. But they are not primitive. They can move, eat, eliminate waste, defend against enemies, and reproduce with remarkable efficiency.

Microbes in the second domain, Archaea, are single-cell organisms that look very much like bacteria under a microscope but have unique ways of making a living. They stem from a different branch on the tree of life, with different genes and biochemistry. Many of them are extremophiles that thrive in environments like boiling hot springs and salty lakes. But others live in milder climates, in the oceans and even in the human gut and skin.

The third domain is the Eukaryota, in which we find the microbes of the Fungi and Protista kingdoms. These Fungi are not toadstools in a forest but a single-celled version of this kind of life. You are undoubtedly familiar with yeasts, valuable for making bread, beer, and wine. But some, such as *Candida*, can also cause unpleasant infections. The Protista are single-celled relatives of plants, animals, and fungi. They are the latest incarnation of our microbial ancestors.

Finally, and somewhat contentiously, we have the viruses. While it's debatable whether they're alive, there's no doubt that they are incredibly efficient at replicating themselves by harvesting the cellular machinery of cells around them.

Collectively, these microbiota—the bacteria, archaea, fungi, protists, and viruses—constitute the microbiome of a particular plant, animal, or ecosystem.

Another mind-boggling fact is that all these invisible microbes outweigh all visible life by a factor of 100 million. Collectively they are heavier than all the plants and animals—all the whales, elephants, and rain forests—that you can see around you.

Visible life is overwhelmingly composed of eukaryotes—single cells that contain a nucleus and that evolved over the last 600 million years into everything big. You are a eukaryote because the cells that make up your body are eukaryotic. Yet unlike microbial eukaryotes, which only have a single cell, your body is made up of tens of trillions of cells that have differentiated into all the different body parts—each of which still has your genetic code locked in its nucleus. As we'll see in Chapter 2, collectively, your eukaryotic cells have developed many special relationships with microbes.

But before we get to the human microbiome, let us entertain you with some of the more hostile habitats that microbes call home.

Bacteria and archaea have been discovered living in Martian-like conditions on volcanoes in South America, with no water, extreme temperatures, and intense levels of ultraviolet light. They extract energy and carbon from wisps of gases flowing from Earth's interior.

The oceans contain at least 20 million kinds of marine microbes that make up 50 to 90 percent of the ocean's biomass. There is a mat of bacteria on the seafloor off the west coast of South America that covers an area roughly the size of Greece. Mud pulled from more than five thousand feet below the seafloor off Newfoundland was found to be teeming with microbes.

Bacteria at hydrothermal vents inhabit everything—rocks, the seafloor, and the insides of mussels and tube worms. They thrive in highly acidic, alkaline, or salty boiling water under high pressure and heat. Some heat-loving thermophiles grow at

235 degrees Fahrenheit. They lend the deep blue, green, and orange colors to Yellowstone's boiling ponds.

Microbes dwell in the rocks found in the world's deepest gold mines. In fact, they can "eat" gold, sequestering it like Lilliputian miners.

Recently, a new genus of bacteria, *Candidatus frackibacter*, has been found living inside hydraulic fracturing wells in Appalachian Basin shale beds. Similarly, acid-loving microbes make their home in mine drainage sites.

After the *Deepwater Horizon* oil spill in the Gulf of Mexico in 2010, microbes gorged themselves on oil and natural gas. They chewed through a toxic stew of hydrocarbons.

Microbes eat plastic. As much as 8 million metric tons of the stuff are dumped into our oceans every year. Trouble is, each piece of plastic takes at least 450 years to decompose. The Great Pacific Garbage Patch, a floating vortex of plastic waste far out to sea, is home to about a thousand different kinds of microbes living on the debris. Landfills contain mountains of polyethylene terephthalate, a plastic used to make water bottles, salad spinners, and peanut butter jars. While it's the most recycled plastic in the United States, two-thirds of it escape our household bins. Researchers recently screened 250 samples of sediment, soil, wastewater, and sludge to see if any microbe might like to eat the plastics. One volunteered: *Ideonella sakaiensis*.

They even munch uranium. Fungi have been deployed to absorb radiation from tainted water at the Fukushima nuclear reactor in Japan.

Some bugs make their living forty miles high up in the sky. In the upper atmosphere, they help form clouds, snow, and rain. When raindrops land on the leaves of trees and shrubs, the bacteria within them can cause water to freeze, creating ice crystals even when they wouldn't form otherwise. These crystals damage plant tissues, allowing the microbes to get inside. Once there the microbes can exploit the resources of the plant (of course the plant thinks of this as an infection!).

Bacteria can survive in space. They rode in all the space shuttles and are ensconced in the International Space Station. The Russians exposed microbes to space for a year, outside of the *Mir* space station, and some survived. NASA scientists suspect that water channels emerge sporadically on Mars and would like Curiosity, the robotic rover that is tooling around, exploring the terrain on Mars, to take a look. But since the rover may carry Earth's microbes, which would thrive rapidly in the water, they can't take the chance of getting too close for fear of contaminating this off-world water source.

They also live closer to home. Extremophiles have been found in dishwashers, hot-water heaters, washing machine bleach dispensers, and hot tubs. They are on every household surface and even in your tap water. We harness them to make food, drugs, alcohol, perfumes, and fuel. Nearly every antibiotic is derived from microbes.

And if all this isn't enough, they eat you when you die.

2

The Human Microbiome

As you saw in Chapter 1, Earth has its own microbiome. It's everywhere—in soil, air, water, forests, mountains, fracking fluids, gold mines, and hot-water heaters.

But animals have their own microbiome, and like you and your child, they acquire it at birth from their mothers, other animals, and the environment. Baby Komodo dragons share their skin and mouth microbes with their surroundings. Octopus eggs are colonized by friendly bacteria within hours of being fertilized. Vampire bats and koala babies acquire microbes from their mothers that allow them to digest their highly specialized diets.

Every creature has coevolved with its own collection of bugs. Termites can digest wood only because of the bacteria in their guts, which break down the otherwise indigestible cellulose. Cows absorb nutrients from grass thanks to the microbes living in their four stomachs. Aphids depend so heavily on their gut microbes that they have delegated the ability to produce essential nutrients like amino acids to their bacteria. Aphids no longer have the genes to carry out these functions. Their microbes do.

Humans have a microbiome too. Perhaps you've read that

there are ten times as many microbes in your body as there are human cells. Unfortunately, that ratio came from a back of the envelope estimate made in 1972, and because it was such a compelling image, it stuck. A more recent analysis puts the ratio at 1.3 microbes per human cell.[1] Thus an average guy will have about 40 trillion bacterial cells and 30 trillion human cells. Individual differences in body size and gender skew the ratio, but you get the idea: we are a superorganism. You harbor about ten thousand microbial species that altogether weigh about three pounds—the same as your brain.

Recall the definition of a microbiome. It is all the microbes and all the genes acting in concert.

Here, microbes have the upper hand. There are at least one hundred microbial genes for every human gene, and they are responsible for many of the biochemical activities associated with your body, ranging from digesting carbohydrates in your food to making some of your vitamins.

Importantly, the microbiome is the genome that you can and do change every day. Although our human genome is fixed our whole lives, the genes in our microbiomes change in response to our food, our environment, drugs we take, and even our health. And at no time is this truer than in early childhood.

Our goal in doing research is to learn how to tweak the microbiome to enhance human health. And this raises a critical issue. From birth to age three, your child's microbiome, especially in the gut, is extremely dynamic. It changes day to day, week to week, following a general pattern that acquires microbes, catch as catch can.

By age three, your toddler's microbiome will have assumed an adult-like pattern. It is mostly stable and tends to bounce back after challenges. All the key microbial players are there, having taken up residence in all the moist and dry niches of your child's body. There they stay, fending off pathogens, breaking down fibers, tuning the immune system, and even influencing mental health.

Thus the first three years of life are profoundly important. Interventions in the very young can have the largest and most lasting effects on health and disease. Although some things that happen in the first three years are beyond your (or anyone's) control, the people your child interacts with, the foods they eat, the places they go, and the medications they take can have lifelong effects. What they encounter in those early years serves as a critical inoculation for their wellbeing.

This is why dirt is so good. It exposes your child to a huge array of harmless germs that, while they may not colonize us, have complex traits to train up your

While we use the terms "good bacteria" and "bad bacteria" in this book, we don't mean it literally. Think of dark chocolate: it can be good or bad depending on how much you eat, and on what else you're eating. Bacteria are shape-shifters, existing as a continuum of lifestyles, not fixed categories. They can assume goodness or badness, conferring health or even death, based on environmental conditions and specific gene interactions. For example, *E. coli* is harmless in most people's gut, but it occasionally causes problems ranging from diarrhea to urinary tract infections. Even the bacterium that causes typhoid fever doesn't harm most of the people it infects. In many people, meningitis bacteria are carried harmlessly in the back of the nose and throat. But one in a hundred or one in a thousand other people can become infected via close personal contact with a carrier. We have even found that some of the bacteria that are considered to be beneficial in your gut can, when stressed, turn to the dark side and infect your body's tissues.

Remember, your body is designed to keep bacteria in the right places. Like a shepherd, the immune system keeps beneficial bacteria close, but not too close. Some of those "good" bacteria will consume your corpse. Similarly, if you give them half a chance now, they'll have a go at it while you're alive. Like people, the same bacteria can be good or bad depending on the context, including the strain, the environment, and the host.

baby's immune system. Many people think that an activated immune system, with lots of inflammation, is good, but in fact the reverse is true. A well-trained immune system damps down inflammation when it's not needed, just as a highly trained athlete's heart races during exercise but has a low pulse the rest of the time.

Microbes can come from the strangest places. Rob recalls a friend who said, "The weirdest part of being a mom is saying sentences I never thought I could imagine, like 'Never put your finger in that part of the kitty.'"

Think for a moment about our evolutionary history. We evolved as hunter-gatherers and early agriculturalists. Our world was filled with dirt, animals, and wild foods we had to hunt or collect. We've only cleaned things up in the last couple of hundred years.

Your baby comes into the world with a biological program expecting to see conditions similar to that past. You can help by providing missing pieces in a commonsense manner. And that is what the rest of this book is all about.

3

Pregnancy

Can my microbiome affect my ability to conceive? Are bacteria related to infertility?

We often get asked these questions. Trying to conceive can be difficult. Everyone wants to know why things are not just happening as they should. Unfortunately, right now there is very little data that could support a solid answer. As we often say, this is a topic of active research.

Examples of this active research include testing to find out whether bacterial vaginosis (BV)—growth of less common kinds of bacteria in the vagina—is related to infertility—and whether it interferes with conception and early pregnancy after in vitro fertilization.[1]

BV is extremely common. Symptoms include a white or gray vaginal discharge with a fishy smell. It usually does not itch or burn. The risk of contracting a sexually transmitted disease such as HIV doubles when you have an active BV infection (although the picture is less clear if you simply have an unusual vaginal microbiome). BV has also been associated with premature birth, a topic being researched in Jack's lab, but no causal link has yet been identified.

BV is caused by an imbalance in vaginal microbes, particularly a reduction in lactobacilli. Women who douche frequently are especially prone to it. So trying to keep the vagina "too clean" in the short run can lead to problems in the long run. The consensus medical advice is that the drawbacks of douching greatly outweigh the benefits. And these drawbacks range from problems conceiving to cervical cancer.

A meta-analysis of twenty-three studies exploring conception, loss of an embryo, or later miscarriage found that BV was correlated with loss of an embryo within the first few weeks of a pregnancy. The infection made the embryo less able to implant itself effectively in the wall of the uterus, one of the earliest steps toward a successful pregnancy. Inflammation may be a factor, but exactly how BV causes inflammation is not known.[2] However, if you're diagnosed with BV and trying to get pregnant, it is often treatable with antibiotics.

However, the link between inflammation and infertility is well known. For example, chlamydia, a sexually transmitted disease, is associated with infertility, especially in women whose pelvic symptoms are left untreated, and can also infect the newborn. When *Chlamydia* and human cell lines are grown on a petri dish in the lab and an inflammation-suppressing probiotic called *Lactobacillus crispatus* is added, the *Chlamydia* cells no longer stick to the human cells. This suggests that pathogenic infections that cause inflammation and lead to infertility can be interrupted by good bacteria.

Women who routinely lose embryos early in pregnancy are thought to be infertile, but their vaginal microbiome and level of inflammation may be to blame. The hope is that in the future we can find ways to dampen these inflammatory events. One could even imagine applying yogurt, either with naturally occurring *Lactobacillus* or with new probiotic strains, to the vagina while trying to conceive. The semen of fertile men has also been shown to have a greater abundance of *Lactobacillus* in a small association study.[3] We have no evidence that this could work, and we certainly don't recommend applying yogurt to the vagina or the penis during sex, but it's the type of idea that could one day lead to a new treatment. You'd want to see how it performs in clinical trials before trying it yourself.

Can my partner's microbiome affect my fetus?

Great question, no data. In principle the answer is yes because your microbiome can affect your fetus and you exchange microbes with your partner. Couples trade all sorts of bacteria, so they tend to look more microbiologically similar because they share intimacy and space.[4] But just sharing space with someone—in an office, for example—does not mean that your microbiomes will become as similar as those of two people who are physically interacting and living together, such as you and your partner. (Interestingly, couples who live with a dog tend to look more similar to each other than do couples without a dog.[5] So if you're wondering if getting a dog brings you closer together, the answer is yes, at least in terms of your microbiomes.)

But on the whole, just because you are swapping germs doesn't mean that the microbes that you're sharing could affect your fetus. Obviously, sexually transmitted diseases can influence the success of your pregnancy and even cause preterm birth. But there have been no studies that have asked the question, does increased microbial sharing between a couple influence the fetus (in either a good or bad way)? You might equally imagine that having a partner with a particularly good microbiome might transmit some good microbes to your fetus, but again there's no evidence. So snuggle up. It can't hurt and you'll have some good times.

Should I visit a dentist before getting pregnant?

Yes, it's a good idea to get a checkup. If you have poor oral health, you may be plagued by mouth sores or bleeding gums. These can allow oral bacteria to enter your bloodstream and stick to the membranes inside your arteries, making it easier for them to cross these membranes.[6] This can allow other bacteria, including harmful pathogens, to invade your bloodstream.[7]

Once in your blood, bacteria can make their way to the membranes surrounding your baby, which are part of your placenta, and cause an infection called chorioamnionitis.[8] Doctors used to think that the offending bacteria only came from a woman's genital tract, but recent research suggests that they may also come from her mouth. Some of these do no harm and don't even have the genes that are involved in causing disease. But when pathogens are in the mix, preterm labor and birth can result.[9]

So far, this route of infection is more hypothetical than proven fact. Studies that look for bacteria originating in the mouth in placental tissue find scant evidence that they are there. What has been detected when tissues are analyzed could be contamination from another source. Clinical trials aimed at improving oral health in pregnant women to reduce the likelihood of premature birth have not found any benefit,[10] although maybe these trials have been carried out too late in pregnancy. If you have chronic poor oral health, it's possible that harmful bacteria could be circulating in your bloodstream long before your placenta develops.[11]

The takeaway is that if you plan on getting pregnant, you should consider visiting your dentist to make sure your oral health is good. And you'll have a better-looking smile.

Are GMOs safe to eat while pregnant? Are organic foods better than conventionally grown foods?

Like nearly all scientists, we feel that genetically modified organisms are safe to eat. Based on all that we know, there's no plausible way that GMO foods could exert an effect—good or bad—on your microbiome. Moreover, nearly every crop and animal food we consume has already been modified from its wild-type state. As far as the evidence shows, foods that have been manipulated in the laboratory to produce transgenic strains are as safe as those produced by more traditional breeding methods (including radiation, which has been widely used since the 1920s to produce new crops through mutation). While some people worry that GMOs could pass genes into their microbiome, the probability of your bacteria acquiring genes through transient exposure to a plant or animal through modified food is essentially nil.

The major criticisms aimed at these foods are environmental and political, which is beyond the scope of this book. The controversy is also highly emotional. When talking about pregnancy and childbirth, people tend to want absolute guarantees of safety. Of course, that's impossible, but we're not talking about logic. We can jabber all day long about safety trials that support GMOs, but critics will shoot back that we don't have all the evidence or we are ignoring theirs. It comes down to a wavering trust in academic science and a deep mistrust of corporations like Monsanto. You'll need to decide for yourself.

You might also wonder if eating organic food will make your pregnancy healthier or improve the quality of your breast milk. We have no evidence that it will. Stanford University researchers carried out a meta-analysis on organic and conventionally grown foods.[12] A meta-analysis is a statistical approach that combines results from multiple studies to resolve uncertainties and reveal the strongest evidence. Based on forty years of research, it concluded that fruits and vegetables labeled organic were, on average, no more nutritious than their conventional and less expensive counterparts. Nor were they any less likely to be contaminated by dangerous bacteria like *E. coli*. Conventional fruits and vegetables did have more pesticide residues, but the levels were always below safety limits set by the Environmental Protection Agency.

But the study, which mainly focused on nutritional value, found other reasons for mothers to consider organic produce (if they can afford it). Three studies identified pregnant women exposed to relatively high amounts of pesticides (known as organophosphates) and then followed their children for years. In elementary school, those children had, on average, slightly lower IQs compared to their peers. (See Chapter 8 for more information on this topic.)

Can microbes explain my food cravings? Why pickles and ice cream at night?

Yes, but we need more studies to show exactly how. Pregnant women experience extreme hormonal changes during pregnancy. For example, progesterone levels increase nearly tenfold and drastically decrease after delivery. These roller-coaster changes have been implicated in depressive disorders. But we believe they can also affect your food cravings.[13]

Here's what we know so far. Changes in your hormone levels can influence your gut environment, which leads to changes in your immune system. That in turn can change the composition and structure of your microbiome.[14] While these interactions occur on many levels, it's entirely plausible that they underlie your food cravings during pregnancy.

We have somewhat better evidence that your microbiome can play a role in cravings when you are not pregnant. When Jack travels to China, he indulges wholeheartedly in the local fare. Oddly, he always experiences an almost complete cessation of his near-constant cravings for chocolate. What might explain this anecdotal observation?

Well, compared to people who don't crave chocolate, chocolate lovers have gut bacteria that produce metabolites that help drive their passion for Lindt bars.[15] When chocolate hounds travel abroad and change what they eat—say, Chinese food instead of meatballs and spaghetti—both their gut microbes and metabolites are affected. As a result, they may temporarily lose their chocolate cravings. When they return home and start eating their regular diet, the metabolites that hunger for chocolate may bounce back. They certainly do for Jack.

More broadly speaking, some researchers think that food cravings, especially for sugar and fat, could be linked to an evolutionary conflict between your gut microbes and your own health interests. The premise is that gut organisms subtly manipulate your immune, nervous, and hormonal systems to shift their environment in ways that favor their growth. Therefore, a bacterial species that grows really well on simple sugars might induce you to crave sugary foods. Given a regular supply of sugar, they will flourish and multiply, leading to a potential positive-feedback loop: more sugar equals more microbes, which equals more sugar. Hence an inability to resist your cravings, even when you're pregnant, may not be due to your lack of willpower but to the power of your gut microbes to drive you to the ice-cream parlor. However, so far the evidence to support this hypothesis is limited, and much more research needs to be done to make sense of this complex web of interactions.

Are microbes involved in my gaining too much weight in pregnancy?

Yes. Microbes and obesity are intimately linked. Chubby or fat people tend to have gut bacteria that promote or sustain weight gain by extracting more energy from the foods they eat. Lean or skinny people tend to have different gut bacteria that do not extract as much energy. (Who ever said life was fair?) Also, gut bacteria found in overweight folks can actually promote the production of fat tissue, leading to changes in the way energy is regulated in the body. The bacteria do this through a complex interaction between the body's immune system, endocrine system (which governs hormones), and circadian rhythm (time sense).[16] The microbiome changes profoundly during pregnancy, with women in their third trimester having markedly different microbiomes than those in their first trimester. Amazingly, when these microbiomes are transplanted into germ-free mice, only the microbiomes from the third trimester cause the mice to develop insulin resistance and inflammation, which are common in the third trimester but not the first.

Being obese before you get pregnant or gaining too much weight during your pregnancy can increase risks for both you and your baby. For example, a weight gain of more than forty pounds over nine months is associated with an increased risk of neurodevelopmental disorders such as autism. Women who gain excessive weight are less able to absorb folate, which is an essential B vitamin. Lack of folate can lead to birth defects, such as spina bifida, anencephaly, and some heart defects. Moreover, infants born to obese mothers can be abnormally large (leading to increased risk of cesarean or difficult vaginal delivery) and suffer from metabolic disorders such as too much insulin and low blood sugar.

Currently, about two-thirds of American women between the ages of fifteen and forty-five are overweight or obese. Overweight women who become pregnant are six times more likely than lean women to gain too much weight and suffer negative health effects, such as gestational diabetes and preeclampsia. Moreover, a mother's high-fat diet during pregnancy can have a lasting impact on the bacteria found in her baby's gut.[17] Studies show that such infants have fewer microbes from the genus *Bacteroides* than normal after birth, an effect that lasts up to six weeks of age. Since these bacteria are involved in breaking down and extracting energy from certain carbohydrates, especially those found in mother's milk, the babies might not be able to derive energy from food in the normal way. Their immune development may also be thrown off track.

Of course the best (but not easiest) way to address this problem would to change your diet before you get pregnant, to promote the growth of bacteria like those found in lean people. The good news is that, in future, you may be able to help this process along by adding a probiotic to your diet. The bad news is that organisms able to do this have not yet been identified.

Do microbes have a role in gestational diabetes?

Quite possibly. Gestational diabetes is a condition in which previously nondiabetic women are diagnosed with diabetes during their pregnancy.

Diabetes is a group of metabolic diseases marked by high blood sugar over a long period of time. Those afflicted experience intense thirst, hunger, and frequent urination. It is caused when the pancreas does not produce enough insulin—a hormone that promotes the absorption of sugar from the blood—or the body's cells fail to respond properly to insulin.

Gestational diabetes significantly impacts the health of the mother and her fetus, as well as her newborn.[18] Women who experience this type of diabetes have an increased risk of high blood pressure and protein in their urine (preeclampsia), a higher risk of developing type 2 diabetes later on, and a greater likelihood of delivering an abnormally large infant. Their babies can suffer from growth abnormalities (either growing too much or too little), respiratory distress, and low blood sugar at birth. Low blood sugar can cause bluish-colored or pale skin, breathing problems, irritability or listlessness, loose or floppy muscles, poor feeding or vomiting, problems keeping the body warm, tremors, shakiness, sweating, or seizures.

The elevated blood sugar seen in gestational diabetes might also affect fetal brain development (leading to autism), but this has only been seen in preterm infants. Moms with gestational diabetes who deliver closer to full term and those with type 2 diabetes throughout their pregnancy do not show this increased risk.

Normally, when blood sugar rises, insulin-producing cells respond to lower blood sugar. This dynamic balance is critical for your health.

Enter microbes. Recall that some of your gut bacteria ferment fiber to make metabolites called short-chain fatty acids (SCFAs) that are very good for you. (The name is clunky, but, as you will see throughout this book, SCFAs are very important.) Turns out your insulin-producing cells can sense the concentration of SCFAs in your gut. In ways we don't completely understand, pregnancy changes the abundance and type of gut bacteria that make SCFAs. And this exerts an influence on insulin secretion.

Mouse experiments show that if you suppress the bacteria that make SCFAs, the amount of the metabolite falls and the animal has fewer insulin-producing cells.[19] And when a mouse or human does not have enough insulin, diabetes results.

If this proves true in humans, we will need to find ways to increase the abundance of gut bacteria that release SCFAs. Surprisingly, this is not that difficult. We know that we can increase bacterial production of SCFAs in children by feeding them an oral probiotic such as *Lactobacillus rhamnosus* GG (see food allergy section). While we still have to confirm this, the same may be true for adults.

Another approach is to nourish SCFA-producing bacteria. Pregnant women could simply increase their fiber intake. That would fuel the fermentation which leads to SCFA production. This is an active field of research and we expect to have therapies soon— but diet modulation and probiotics are a good place to start.

Does exercise influence my microbiome? Could it help with my pregnancy?

Animal studies suggest that increased exercise alters the microbiome and improves memory—that is, if you're a mouse. But we don't really understand why. It could be that exercise influences the immune system in ways that restructure the gut's microbial community, preferring species that control inflammation. Such microbes also produce chemicals that influence the health of the brain and hormonal system. It's been noted that exercise reduces some bacteria (such as those in the pro-inflammatory Enterobacteriaceae family) and increases others (such as the anti-inflammatory *Ruminococcus*). But beware; we have not done the proper experiments to test whether the anti-inflammatory effects of exercise are due to these changes in the microbiome.

Whether this link is relevant to humans has not been established. We don't yet know if your level of exercise will affect your gut microbes, whether or not you are pregnant. But the mouse studies have turned up one interesting fact. Forced exercise, as opposed to voluntary exercise, affects the mouse microbiomes differently, particularly with regard to levels of gut inflammation.[20] While we don't yet understand how this all works, it's possible that forced exercise could lead to anxiety, which could lead to an elevation of bacteria that induce or fail to prevent gut inflammation.[21] While this is supposition, it does suggest that you should only do as much exercise as you feel comfortable with, while following the advice of your doctor or midwife for exercise during your pregnancy. But on the whole a little exercise may help change your microbiome and reduce inflammation, which is all to the good. And if you can get outside, you will likely feel better for it.

Are microbes responsible for premature birth?

Yes, sometimes, but it's complicated. Most causes of preterm birth do not involve microbes and range from exposures to chemicals in the environment to medical conditions or genetics.

However, as mentioned earlier, if you develop a bacterial infection in your vagina during your pregnancy, you stand a greater likelihood of going into preterm labor and experiencing a premature birth. Preterm labor means you will experience contractions every ten minutes, or more frequently, before your thirty-seventh week, and sometimes as early as your twenty-seventh week of pregnancy. Your newborn may weigh less than two pounds and face a lifetime of health challenges, including underdeveloped lungs, problems with sight and hearing, and possibly cerebral palsy and later developmental delays.

In some cases, an antibiotic treatment aimed at the bacterial infection will prevent a premature birth, suggesting that vaginal pathogens may play a role in triggering the condition.

But here's where it gets complicated. Many women experience preterm labor contractions that do not lead to a premature birth—and yet they have the same vaginal infections as women who do. We don't know why, although we know it is a complex relationship between inflammation and how close the pathogens get to the placenta. What we do know is that preterm labor contractions are very common and that they resolve in the majority of women.

A number of risk factors related to preterm labor and premature birth include having had a prior preterm birth, having an extremely high or low body weight, a pregnancy with multiple fetuses (twins, triplets, etc.), stress, as well as lack of dental and prenatal care.[22] Doctors don't yet understand why these factors lead to premature labor, but we do know that many of them are linked to increased inflammation.

Bacteria are also implicated in premature birth.[23] As noted in the entry on infertility, vaginal infections can interfere with and terminate an early pregnancy. But until recently, there has been scant evidence that such infectious microbes can cross into the placenta and infect the fetus. The placenta is thought to be an impervious barrier, at least to most bacteria.

A recent study upended the privileged status of the placenta when it found that a common vaginal infection, group B streptococcus (GBS), can lead to preterm and stillbirths in mice.[24] Not surprisingly, these bacteria prompted inflammation in the mouse mother's body, including the placenta. But when researchers looked closely, they saw no signs of the GBS bacteria in the placenta. Then a deeper look revealed a surprise. The mother's vagina, which was colonized with GBS, had sent little packets of inflammation across the placenta and into the womb.

Whether this alarming phenomenon of dangerous microbes reaching the fetus holds true for humans is not known. But if you have a GBS infection while you are pregnant, prompt treatment with antibiotics seems advisable. However, one in four women are colonized with GBS during pregnancy, and whether antibiotics are needed for these asymptomatic GBS infections is much less clear.

A related issue is asymptomatic bacteriuria (bacteria in the urine with no apparent discomfort). This is typically treated with antibiotics to reduce the risk of preterm labor or delivery. However, emerging evidence that a natural urinary microbiome exists may lead to a reevaluation of whether antibiotics should automatically be used.

Before we move on to other topics, we'd like to warn you about a little-known downside of certain antibiotics. The medicine you take to fight a bacterial infection can harm your baby—at least according to a recent study in mice. In an experiment, pregnant animals were infected with *Streptococcus pneumoniae,* which can lead to pneumonia, ear infections, and bacterial meningitis in humans. When researchers treated the mice with ampicillin, a commonly prescribed antibiotic, the bacteria were destroyed when the drug burst their cell walls.

Surprisingly, pieces of the broken cell walls were observed crossing the mouse placenta and entering immature neurons, causing them to proliferate via a previously unrecognized pathway. After birth, the infant animals had memory problems and impaired cognitive functioning. Although this was a study in animals, the same mechanism might underlie the association between human bacterial infections during pregnancy and an increased risk of autism and other cognitive problems in children.

The take-home message here is that pregnant women should consider requesting antibiotics that kill bacteria without bursting their cell walls. However, some of these antibiotics, such as tetracycline, can have other effects such as harming fetal tooth and bone development. We recommend that you talk with your doctor to balance the risks and benefits during antibiotic selection.

Lest we leave you thinking that bacteria are natural-born baby killers, we'd like to tell you about other kinds of microbes that pump out metabolites—chemicals that result from biological activity—that quite literally calm down your immune system and dampen inflammation. Their names are not all that important, but their activity can play an important role in your pregnancy.

Preliminary evidence from Jack's lab suggests that women who experience preterm labor and premature birth are likely to have less of the kinds of bacteria that produce immune-calming short-chain fatty acids. The bacteria that produce these helpful chemicals are those that ferment fiber in your gut.

If our observation is true, it's likely that anything that increases the abundance of fiber-munching bacteria in your gut could also leave you less susceptible to inflammation and preterm labor. How to do this? It's simple. Eat more fiber, especially whole grains, leafy vegetables, and fruit, and your gut will take care of the rest. It will start making more metabolites that help control inflammation, as well as promoting overall health, as shown in too many studies to list. Also, you could help this along by avoiding simple sugars and complex starches that promote the growth of pro-inflammatory bacteria.

Currently there is next to no evidence that this strategy will reduce the risks of premature birth,[25] but since eating a healthy diet during pregnancy is recommended, it wouldn't be a bad thing to try, especially if you have the risk factors we mentioned.

What can cross my placenta?

Both good things and bad. The placenta is a complex and poorly understood organ that anchors your fetus to your uterus, nourishing your infant and providing a barrier to any harmful bacteria, fungi, parasites, and viruses that may invade your body.

Traditionally, the placenta is viewed as an impermeable barrier to bacteria and parasites. It separates your experience from your fetus's sterile environment. Remember, however, that viruses are also part of the microbiome, and they are so small that they can easily slip through this barrier. So we have evolved a defense mechanism. Placental cells (called trophoblasts) can sense viruses and call for help when there is an invasion. They release molecules that summon immune cells to come and clear out viral infection. It's a wonderful solution that works most of the time. Unfortunately, some viruses can fight back by promoting chronic inflammation and triggering trophoblasts to commit mass suicide. Thus the fetus remains vulnerable to the virus. This scenario has been linked to the development of autism-like symptoms in mice and a variety of birth defects.

Some of the best-known viruses that can outmaneuver your placenta's protective mechanisms include rubella (German measles), cytomegalovirus, HIV, and the newly notorious Zika virus.

Rubella is a mild disease marked by a low-grade fever, swollen lymph nodes, and rash. When a mother is infected in her first trimester, her baby may suffer a variety of birth defects, including eye problems, heart defects, hearing loss, microcephaly, bone disease, mental retardation, and diabetes. All pretty serious, which is why a vaccine was first licensed in 1969.

Cytomegalovirus (CMV) is a common infection that can cross through the placenta and infect the fetus. Most infants with congenital CMV infections never show signs or have health problems, but some can develop hearing and/or mental coordination problems later in life. If a child is adversely affected, doctors can prescribe antiviral medications. There is no way to categorically screen for CMV infection, and currently there is no vaccine.

HIV exacts a different toll. Most babies born to HIV-infected mothers surprisingly do not acquire infection, but they experience twice the mortality of children born to HIV-negative mothers. Why? According to a recent study, the mother's HIV infection insidiously changes the microbiome of her uninfected infant. The baby will have very different strains and abundances of key bacterial species (such as *Prevotella* and *Pseudomonas*), their guts will be inflamed, and their mother's milk will show unusual microbial communities.

The placenta is also a poor and ineffective barrier against certain parasites. One of the most common, *Toxoplasma gondii*, is found in cat poop. When pregnant women scoop up cat litter and accidentally breathe in the particles, the parasite can find its way to their placentas. Like viruses, it can damage placental cells and cause them to commit suicide. The resulting condition, called toxoplasmosis, can lead to fetal infection, miscarriage, congenital disease, or disability later in life. This is why many pregnant women get their partners to empty the cat box for nine months.

The latest threat to infant health is the mosquito-borne Zika virus. It can cross the placenta in every trimester and cause birth defects, particularly unusually small heads, or microcephaly. Estimates are that more than 1.6 million childbearing women in the Americas could become infected in coming years. Based on published models, tens of thousands of pregnancies could be affected. The virus is spreading throughout the Western Hemisphere and Asia. In August 2016, it was found in Puerto Rico, and Miami, Florida.

The virus is spread by mosquitoes, most commonly those of the genus *Aedes*. But it can also spread through sexual intercourse, as well as through saliva and tears. The Zika virus can persist for months in semen, and, in what came as a surprise to researchers, it can spread from an infected woman to a man during sex.

How the virus enters the brain of a developing fetus is an urgent question. It's likely to be by the same mechanisms as the other viruses mentioned above—by causing the host's immune system to turn against itself. But in July 2016 researchers showed that Zika can infect several types of placental cells, including macrophages. It may invade via multiple routes, such as creeping though tiny openings, hitching a ride on an antibody, or binding to proteins on placental cells. From there it can access the amniotic fluid and even the brain of the fetus. We still have much to learn about this nasty virus.

. . . .

Thankfully, good stuff can also pass through your placenta to help your unborn baby. Your immune system, acting in concert with friendly microbes, can give your baby a head start.[26] Well, again, this has only been shown in mice, but we're hopeful that the biology will generalize to us humans.

Let's look at another experiment. When pregnant mice were exposed to low levels of nonpathogenic or good *E. coli* (not the notorious bacteria that caused food poisoning at Chipotle restaurants), their pups had more immune cells to fight infection and fewer immune cells that promote inflammation. Basically, their immune systems had been ramped up, readying the pups for the tsunami of microbes that would colonize them at birth. So far so good.

But here's a surprise. The bacteria were not the direct cause of this boost. Instead, they joined forces with a variety of gut microbes to produce metabolites that made their way through the mother's body to her placenta and into her milk. Pups exposed to these metabolites were better off, with higher levels of important immune factors and a healthier gut lining.

Can the use of antibiotics during pregnancy affect my infant?

Potentially yes. Using antibiotics during pregnancy, although often life-saving and important when medically indicated, has been linked to metabolic and immune diseases in infants and older children.[27] The basic premise is that taking these drugs risks disrupting the diversity and abundance of microbes that you transfer to your baby during a vaginal delivery.[28] That is not a good thing.

For example, children born to mothers who took antibiotics during their second and third trimesters had an 84 percent higher risk of obesity at age seven compared with children whose mothers did not take antibiotics.[29] Another study found that the number of days a woman takes an antibiotic while pregnant correlates with an increased risk of persistent wheezing (a precursor for asthma) or other allergic diseases in her child.[30]

Antibiotics that alter your gut microbiome during pregnancy may affect your developing fetus in other ways as well.[31] Bacteria, or at least chemicals that they produce, can circulate in the bloodstreams of some pregnant women and cross into their placentas. We have yet to do the proper studies to confirm this, but these chemicals may influence how your fetus develops. What's puzzling is that the changes that can occur are very broad. For example, antibiotic disruption of your microbiome during pregnancy could lead to an increase in pro-inflammatory markers circulating in your blood, which in turn could negatively affect your baby's development. On the other hand, it's possible that the same sort of antibiotic disruption could lead to the production of more beneficial chemicals, such as short-chain fatty acids or neurotransmitters. The problem is that right now we just don't know which is more likely under what circumstances. One thing is certain. If you are really sick with an infection while you're pregnant, the infection may seriously harm your baby, so please don't forgo medically necessary antibiotics. Ask your physician about possible negative consequences.

Can I take antidepressants while I'm pregnant? Can I take them while I'm nursing?

According to the Centers for Disease and Control and Prevention (CDC), among more than three hundred thousand U.S. women who delivered babies in 2013, about 10 percent suffered from major depression during their pregnancy. Many women don't seek adequate treatment for depression because they fear the social disapproval still associated with the use of antidepressants, or they are afraid of what these drugs may do to their fetus. But failing to treat serious depression can also harm both the mother and fetus. Unfortunately, there is a lack of clear information about the effects of perinatal depression and antidepressants on the fetus and nursing baby.

The most commonly prescribed antidepressants given to pregnant women and new mothers are a class of drugs known as selective serotonin reuptake inhibitors, or SSRIs. You've probably heard of Prozac? It was one of the first SSRIs, typically recommended for anxiety, obsessive compulsive disorder, and depression. To understand how SSRIs work, we need to take a closer look at how the neurotransmitter serotonin behaves in the brain.

To communicate, neurons use neurotransmitters like serotonin to send and receive signals. But neurons do not touch each other directly; instead, information flows from one neuron to another neuron across a synapse—a tiny cleft separating them. When an electric signal travels down an axon (the neuron's main cable), it goes to an area called the presynaptic terminal where neurotransmitters are made and packaged into tiny droplets called vesicles. Then action: the electric charge releases (in this example) serotonin into the cleft, where it scoots over to the postsynaptic cell and binds to serotonin receptors. The molecules fit like keys in a lock. The receiving cell then releases its own electric charge.

But let's go back to the cleft, where it's cleanup time. Any serotonin left over gets destroyed by enzymes or transported back into the presynaptic cell. It's called reuptake. But imagine you want to delay this process. You want more serotonin to reach the postsynaptic cell to keep messages moving. This is what Prozac does. It blocks the reuptake of serotonin and decreases the number of postsynaptic receptors. This inhibition in some unknown way decreases symptoms of depression. Other factors are also involved, such as changes in how the immune system responds to stimuli, and an increase in another important molecule called brain-derived neurotrophic factor (BDNF).

Now, what about microbes? Serotonin, BDNF, and immune pathways interact by changing the gut environment and selecting for different species, so it's reasonable to expect that SSRIs will alter the microbiome. Furthermore, SSRIs are known to have some antimicrobial activity and are associated with the development of metabolic disorders like type 2 diabetes.

We know that gut bacteria make a precursor of serotonin, 5-HT, which, when disrupted, may lead to mental health disorders. But we are just starting to research whether SSRIs alter the microbiome and the potential consequences of such changes. What we do know is that the side effects associated with SSRIs are often associated with microbiome disturbance.

It's shocking how little we know about the effects of antidepressants on women and the fetus both during pregnancy and postpartum.[32] The depression itself and the drugs used to treat it can have negative effects on a developing fetus, including physical and mental disorders and preterm labor.

So if you are depressed, should you take antidepressants during pregnancy and after your baby is born? Well, you need to discuss this with your health professional. The risks and benefits of taking these drugs—or not taking them—depend on a huge number of factors, including your personal history. During pregnancy, it's true that antidepressants are associated with small increases in risk of birth defects, miscarriage, premature birth, and other neonatal complications. However, without treatment, you could develop a major psychological disorder that could interfere with your ability to care for your baby. On the other hand, untreated depression during pregnancy can directly affect the fetus. After delivery, such babies are often irritable and lethargic, with irregular sleep habits. They may grow into infants who are underweight, slow learners, and emotionally unresponsive, with behavior problems such as aggression. Again, talk to your doctor. Unless there is a clear reason to avoid an antidepressant, the medication may be the most appropriate strategy.

Of course there are other ways to help alleviate the symptoms of depression, including exercise, diet, meditation, and counseling. They are worth trying. And we have early evidence, described later, that probiotics can help treat depression. Ongoing work in Jack's lab shows that some bacteria can substantially alleviate depressive behavior in animals. We hope to soon have more focused therapeutic strategies to address these complex conditions.

Our most important message is that you need to take care of yourself. After your baby is born, you should absolutely consider taking an antidepressant. The known side effects greatly outweigh the huge impact that a mental health disorder could have on you and your family. As you are about to undertake the care of a most vulnerable person, antidepressant medications may help transform two lives for the better.

4

···

Birth

Should I give birth at home or in the hospital?

It depends on your circumstances. Jack's first son, Dylan, was born in a hospital under rather complex circumstances. So when it came to planning the birth of his second child, Hayden, Jack and his wife, Kat, opted for a home delivery to help ensure that their baby was delivered vaginally. At the time, home births were being encouraged in the United Kingdom with highly trained midwives and other medical professionals provided by the National Health Service. That experience was wonderful. Kat was in her own bed and within thirty minutes of the birth was breast-feeding a healthy baby boy and eating toast and drinking her favorite English Breakfast tea (decaffeinated, of course!).

Some studies show that complication rates for low-risk births are lower at home than in hospitals.[1] Nearly a third of babies born in hospitals in the United States are delivered via cesarean section, often due to the cautionary nature of modern obstetrical practice.[2] Among seventeen thousand home births in a recent study conducted by the Midwives Alliance of North America, only 5.2 percent needed to go the hospital for a C-section.[3]

The rest were born safely and comfortably at home, although pregnant women who choose to use midwives are likely to be a self-selecting healthy population. According to midwives and their supporters, your odds of delivering a microbially healthy baby are better at home. Two Canadian studies found the same thing.[4] Yet another study showed no significant difference in infections between home and hospital births, with a trend toward fewer such problems in home births.[5]

On the other hand, a study published in the *American Journal of Obstetrics and Gynecology* asserts that the risk of death from all causes is much greater for home births than for hospital births.[6] The best data in this study came from births in Oregon in 2012: the death rate that year for babies in planned home births with a midwife was about seven times that of births at a hospital. The researchers say other studies found perinatal death rate at least triple for home versus hospital.

Here we can offer solid advice. The most important factor in birth outcomes was whether the home birth had been overseen by a certified nurse midwife (CNM) or by a certified professional midwife (CPM). The former are highly qualified (as are those in the UK and Canada), while the latter need only very basic training—essentially, a high school diploma. We therefore recommend that if you are considering a home birth you ensure that you get the services of a certified *nurse* midwife.

The bottom line? The evidence on whether home or hospital is a better place to give birth remains contested. For those in a low-risk category, the trend favors home births because of the reduced rate of C-section and the increased exposure to beneficial microbes. If you're in a high-risk category, however, the additional support that the hospital environment provides can be life-saving.

I had a C-section. I've heard that it may not be good for my baby. What's going on?

First, we want to assure you that C-sections are not inherently bad. In fact, they can be life-saving for both you and your baby, and in developing countries lack of access to C-sections is an important medical issue. Your doctor may recommend the surgery if there are problems with your placenta and a danger of excessive bleeding during a vaginal birth. If you have an infection like HIV or genital herpes, you may want to avoid putting your baby through the birth canal because they may pick up these infections during delivery. Any chronic health condition can lead your doctor to recommend a C-section because vaginal birth puts such great stress on the body.

And then there are complications during labor and birth. Maybe the baby is too big to pass through the birth canal or has turned in a breech or transverse position. Maybe your labor is too slow or it has stopped when it should not. Perhaps the fetus is in distress; its heart rate has slowed, putting it at risk of oxygen deprivation. Or the umbilical cord may collapse or be compressed in such a way that the baby is endangered. We mention these reasons so you won't feel guilty if you ever have to choose a C-section. It's better to be safe than sorry.

However, C-section rates are often higher than they need to be. In private hospitals in Brazil, over 80 percent of babies are delivered via C-section. In the United States, it's one in three infants. In addition to the medical reasons discussed, women may choose this method of delivery for scheduling convenience or out of fear of labor pains. It's an individual choice that most physicians will honor.

But C-sections are coming under closer scrutiny because of an unintended consequence. Vaginal births confer essential microbes on a neonate, with long-lasting health impacts. To the best of our knowledge, your baby's first exposure to microbes comes during the birth process: there is some evidence that a healthy placenta can harbor bacteria, but the jury is still out on this question.[7] Personally, we are not convinced; the kinds of bacteria reported in these studies could easily be technical artifacts or the result of bacterial DNA that has associated with the placenta. Bacteria are routinely found in maternal blood and can be associated with her placenta. But the notion of blood-borne microbes invading the placenta is not supported by available data. In contrast, a bacterial infection of amniotic fluid can contribute to preterm birth.

In all likelihood your baby is essentially free of microbes until the birth process begins—and this is why we see differences in those born vaginally or via C-section.

In a vaginal birth, your baby is squeezed for many hours through the birth canal. It's an arduous journey for both mother and baby, and it serves a profoundly important evolutionary purpose. On the way to the outside world, while still attached to the placenta, your newborn is slathered with vaginal microbes as well as bits of fecal matter. (Every woman who has given birth knows this to be true. It's yucky, but that doesn't mean it's not a good thing.) These first microbes, predominately composed of *Lactobacillus* species, enter your baby's mouth, nostrils, and gastrointestinal tract, setting the stage for their microbiome to develop as nature designed it.

Infants delivered via C-section have a different introduction to our microbial world.[8] Once they are surgically removed from the uterus, the first microbes they encounter come from the people and places around them—the parents, doctors, nurses, other people in the room, as well as the walls, the overhead lamps, and the furniture. These are microbes that are mostly found on skin, which are in and of themselves mostly harmless—they're just not the types of microbes that your infant's burgeoning immune system is expecting to see. The types of bacteria your infant expects are those from the vagina, not from skin.

Most babies delivered by C-section turn out fine. The procedure is not some kind of modern medical curse visited upon helpless infants. But the reason you may be worrying about the safety of C-sections has to do with a growing number of reports relating to an increased risk of diseases or conditions linked to a baby's first microbiome. These include asthma, allergies, atopic dermatitis, obesity, diabetes, celiac, irritable bowel syndrome, and even autism.

As mentioned in Rob's story in the introduction, we have been exploring whether babies' microbiomes can be modified after C-section by swabbing them with their mother's vaginal microbes. The technique, called "vaginal seeding," is simple.[9] The mother has their partner (or mom or whomever is with you in the delivery room) insert sterile cotton pads or a tampon into her vagina before the baby is born. Leave it in for an hour if you have time. The cotton will absorb vaginal fluids and associated microbes. After your baby is delivered and examined by the medical team, you simply swab your baby's mouth, nose, face, ears, skin, and perineum with the collected fluids. You give back what modern obstetrics took away.

Critics of this method often warn against infecting your baby with pathogens that may reside in your vagina. But we believe this risk is extremely low in the United States because nearly all women are screened for such pathogens prior to giving birth. If you have been screened and found positive, then vaginal seeding is most certainly a bad idea and you *should not do it*. However, if you have been screened and found negative, then there is no more risk of infection than if your baby was delivered vaginally.

We do note that the American Academy of Pediatrics has recommended that vaginal seeding not be used until more studies showing benefit have been done.

Evidence to date is that we can modify the microbiome of a C-section baby to resemble that of an infant born vaginally for at least a month after delivery. We don't yet have a large enough sample size of children to know how long this protection might last. But a recent study showed that a trifecta of practices—birth by C-section, exposure to antibiotics, and formula feeding—slows infant development and decreases microbial diversity in the first year of life. Whether these short-term changes have life-long consequences for a child's immune function and metabolism is not yet known.

Like everything involving the microbiome, the findings are complicated. For example, the researchers that performed the vaginal seeding study above found that, compared to vaginally born infants, C-section babies' microbiomes showed significantly greater species diversity—which is sometimes considered a good thing—in the first weeks after birth. But then these measures declined during their first month and continued to fall up to age two. Their microbial diversity failed to mature along the usual pathways. Instead, it stagnated. The change in birth mode interrupted the natural interplay between species diversity and dominance.

A couple of studies that followed cohorts of C-section babies for five years recently reported conflicting results.[10] One, carried out in Scotland, found no long-term health consequences. The other, from Harvard, found that babies born via C-section had 64 percent higher odds of becoming obese compared to their siblings born vaginally.

The jury may be out over the long-term consequences, but it seems prudent to us to avoid C-sections if you have a choice.

Does the vernix have any effect on my baby?

Yes. But not to worry. Since the 1940s, the vernix—the white sticky stuff covering many newborns—has been known to serve as a barrier protecting newborns as they move through the birth canal. A waxy, slippery substance, it serves as moisturizer, anti-infective and antioxidant waterproofing, and wound-healing material. It's also a defense system full of enzymes that combat harmful bacteria.

Despite its protective qualities, the vernix is routinely scrubbed off newborns, presumably because it looks icky and has not seemed all that important. Babies who are washed or bathed after birth don't have higher rates of infections, so it's not immediately apparent that the substance is essential for human health.[11] But babies who get a warm bath instead of a washcloth are calmer and cry less from the cleaning. Some researchers think the vernix could be used as a natural alternative for preparing topical anti-bacterial creams.[12]

Is the microbiome linked to necrotizing enterocolitis?

Yes—but we don't know if it's the cause. Necrotizing entero-colitis, or NEC, is a horrible disease that affects some preterm babies. Essentially, the gut gets infected and then starts to rot from within. The average cost of care for a premature infant with necrotizing enterocolitis is nearly $200,000. The good news is that human breast milk seems to help prevent NEC, reducing the length of hospital stays and costs of caring for the sick babies.

Given what we know about the role of breast milk in shap-ing the developing infant's gut, the microbiome might be in-volved in NEC. In fact, a recent study of 3,586 stool samples from 166 infants—one of the largest infant microbiome projects ever conducted by Phillip Tarr's group at Washington University in St. Louis—showed that changes in the baby's microbiome happen before NEC develops and can even be used to predict the disorder.[13] Specifically, microbes that tend to be more aerobic and faster-growing, such as Gammaproteobacteria, will bloom in advance of NEC, and anaerobic taxa such as *Clostridium* are depleted.[14] The more premature the infant, the clearer this trend.[15]

Although there are dangers in giving live bacteria to extremely premature infants who don't yet have fully developed immune systems, a number of studies have used probiotics to reduce the rates of NEC.[16] Most trials have been successful, achieving about a twofold reduction in incidence.

However, you should know that probiotics can get into a newborn's bloodstream, where they can reproduce wildly and cause problems. So probiotics must be used cautiously under medical supervision. That said, the generally low risks of probiotics versus the severe and debilitating effects of NEC means that we can expect to see them used along with certain antibiotics.

Does birth order affect the microbiome?

Yes. Siblings are protective. In a sample of 606 healthy newborns, the number of older siblings living in the household had a significant effect on the composition and structure of their microbiomes.[17] A child with older siblings was more likely to be colonized at five weeks old with helpful bacteria (such as *Lactobacillus* and *Bacteroides*) and less likely to be colonized with potentially harmful bacteria (such as *Clostridium*).

Interestingly, children who were colonized by *Clostridium* at age five weeks were more likely to develop atopic dermatitis over the next six months of life. This difference persisted for at least thirty-one weeks. It appears that not only do older children help infants become colonized with protective bacteria, but that the benefits last for a long time.

In looking at each child's early life experience, it turns out that much of the protection afforded them came *directly* from older brothers or sisters, the more the better. In large families older kids have been known to poke their snotty fingers into the baby's mouth, sneeze on their rice cereal, or rub dirt into their tiny hands. Importantly, younger siblings are exposed to a wider variety of diseases and microbes that older children drag home from school. All these sources combine to influence the immune system of these younger kids and to structure their microbiome.[18]

The good news is that the high diversity of microbes broadcast by older siblings may help explain the lower allergy risk seen in their younger brothers and sisters.

Do boys and girls have different microbiomes based on the microbes they encounter at birth?

No. As in most things, the sexes are more equal than not. In general, boys and girls don't differ in their microbiomes at birth. Male and female infants begin life mostly microbe-free but rapidly acquire bacteria from the world around them. In newborns, the first bacteria depend on delivery mode: if babies pass through the birth canal, they have mostly vaginal bacteria, but if they are delivered by C-section without any labor, they mostly pick up skin bacteria from the environment. However, they rapidly gain additional bacteria from the people and environment around them—from breast milk, skin-to-skin contact, household dust, and so forth.

Here we need to clarify the distinction between microbiome

and microbiota. The gut microbiota refers to the trillions of microbes inhabiting your intestine. As you age and are exposed to the big wide world, they become quite diverse. Your gut microbiome refers collectively to all the microbes *and their genes*, which code for functions that affect your health.

Studies show that we humans share a functional core microbiome but not core microbiota.[19] In other words, our microbes—the bugs themselves—are different, often wildly different. But the metabolic pathways our microbes use to keep us alive and ticking are very much alike. Many of the genes found throughout the microbial world perform similar routine housekeeping functions. They build cell walls. They replicate. They take out the trash. Each microbe may have its own characteristics and role to play in our world, but they all rely on similar genetic pathways for doing their housework.

Microbes and their genes can be compared to the ecology of rain forests. If viewed from the air, all rain forests look similar, yet they are composed of different species that evolved independently. Your gut is the same. It has functional redundancy, meaning members of the community have similar functional niches and can therefore substitute for one another. In this regard, we have not seen differences between boys and girls.

Adults show no differences in functional diversity (the interactions of all the forest species) but plenty of microbial diversity (many different kinds of trees and plants). However, this diversity is not substantially affected by whether you're male or female. This picture came clear with the Human Microbiome Project, a five-year effort to map the normal microbial makeup of healthy humans. Published in 2012, it "revealed that healthy individuals differ remarkably in the microbes that occupy habitats such as gut, skin and vagina."[20]

The one exception is the urethra, which has different

microbiomes in men and women.[21] This dissimilarity has been observed between the microbiota in male and female voided urine, as well as in urethral swabs. (These are obviously a lot more uncomfortable to collect. In one early study of the microbiome in Rob's lab, researchers originally planned to collect vaginal samples from women and urethral samples from men but dropped this component after it was determined that the male participants couldn't bear to do it more than once—and the study required sampling over time. They did successfully sample twenty-seven other sites, though, which as you can imagine is a lot of places to stick a Q-tip first thing in the morning.)

We find substantial bacterial similarity between the male urethra and female vagina of sexual partners with bacterial vaginosis—a vaginal infection caused by changes in normal bacterial balance. On the other hand, healthy monogamous heterosexual couples have different bacteria in the male urethra and female vagina. But there have been no explicit studies demonstrating urethra compared to urethra. Female samples maintain Actinobacteria and Bacteroidetes bacteria, which are generally absent in men. We don't know when these differences start to occur, in part because we can't ethically obtain samples from the genitals of small children.

However, the American Gut Project based in Rob's lab at the University of California, San Diego, is starting to see subtle differences in the microbiome between men and women when we look at thousands of people. For example, when men and women consume the same amount of saturated fat, women see an increase in *Parabacteroides* whereas men show an increase in *Alistipes*. We don't yet know what these differences mean—just that they are there.

Is there a difference in what microbes come from Mom or Dad?

Another great question and no data. A baby's first microbes naturally come from his or her birth mother during delivery, and then more microbes are transmitted from mother to child during breast-feeding. These early interactions can have profound impacts on a child's microbiome. But, strikingly, no one has performed a study examining the relative impact of fathers on their children's developing microbiomes. There's simply no data on this question, though we do know that children's gut microbiomes resemble those of their mothers and their fathers about equally, even if the adults are stepparents. In other words, the history of shared environmental exposures is more important in shaping gut microbial ecology than biological relatedness. However, we can't yet answer what would happen in most scenarios. For example, if a baby was born vaginally from a birth mother, then adopted as an infant (which can sometimes even include nursing from the mother who was not pregnant), whose microbiome would the infant have? We just don't know.

Of course, fathers must have an impact. When Jack's sons were born, he was ready to embrace the practice of skin bonding. He removed his shirt and hugged both babies to his chest. For Hayden, this occurred a few minutes after his home birth. For Dylan, with his meconium complication, it took longer, about ten minutes after his birth. Either way both his kids received some of his skin and oral bacteria early in life.

Did this transfer influence their microbial makeup? We just don't know. The reason we don't know is that most of the bacteria Jack and his wife share belong to related species, so a simple survey of what microbes are found on his kids' skin can't distinguish which parent the bacteria came from. To get to an answer, we need to dig down deeply into each bacterium's genome and match it to the genomes of the bacterial species found in each parent.

We imagine that if fathers were sole or primary caregivers, their bacteria would predominate in their kids. Same goes for single moms. But when moms and dads raise kids together, along with their dogs, everyone shares the ambient bacteria in the household.[22]

Breast-Feeding

Does it matter if I breast-feed?

You've probably heard people say, "Breast is best." Indeed, many studies show that breast-fed infants have better health outcomes than non-breast-fed infants—fewer ear infections, colds, and bouts of diarrhea. They also have stronger immune systems, score higher in IQ tests, and may be less prone to obesity that other babies. Breast-feeding also has many benefits to mothers, ranging from slimming down more rapidly to release of oxytocin that assists in bonding with your baby, to reduced risks of some kinds of cancers.

But before you embark on a guilt trip about the effects of not breast-feeding on your baby, you should be aware that many of these studies don't fully account for confounding factors. The largest randomized trial ever conducted on the long-term benefits of breast-feeding, carried out in Belarus, Russia, found few demonstrable differences in the children by age six: breast-fed kids were not any healthier than bottle-fed kids.[1] But as babies, breast-fed infants did have fewer colds and other common health problems, so that is something to keep in mind.

What makes breast milk so special?

The answer to this question may surprise you. A major component of your breast milk is not destined to feed your baby. Instead, it is designed to feed the microbes in your infant's gut. It is "food for the bugs."[2] (Although we deal with the concept of prebiotics in other answers, this section provides more detail that you might find useful.)

All mammals make milk, but not all milk is equal. A key ingredient is a menu of complex sugars (called oligosaccharides), and this is where humans stand out. The milk of cows, goats, sheep, and pigs contains oligosaccharide concentrations that are a hundred to a thousand times lower than human milk. No other mammal matches the high amount and high structural diversity of human milk oligosaccharides, called HMOs for short. Human colostrum, the sticky first milk that mothers make, is loaded with HMOs. To date, more than two hundred different HMOs have been identified. They are the third most abundant ingredient in human milk, after lactose and fats. And guess what? Your baby cannot digest them.

Let's assume you are breast-feeding. Your milk contains boatloads of HMOs that travel to your baby's small intestine and colon and go to work feeding bacteria. Acting as prebiotics, they promote and support the growth of good bacteria in your child's gut. (When your baby transitions to solid food, HMOs disappear from their feces.)

One bacterial species is particularly suited to metabolizing the fats, sugars, and proteins found in human milk—*Bifidobacterium longum infantis*, or *B. infantis*. It thrives on HMOs so completely that researchers suggest human milk may have evolved to nourish this one microbe.[3] It dominates the guts of breast-fed infants. And it is a workhorse for keeping your baby healthy.

When *B. infantis* digests HMOs, it releases important metabolites—short-chain fatty acids—that feed certain cells in your baby's gut wall. Those cells, called T regulatory cells, or simply Tregs, regulate your infant's immune system by dialing down and regulating inflammation so it can't spin out of control. This is obviously a critical engine of your child's health, and breast milk is its fuel.

But that's not all. *B. infantis* produces a range of other chemicals and nutrients that help your baby's immune system develop. For example, this microbe encourages infant gut cells to make adhesive proteins that keep other microbes from seeping into your baby's bloodstream. And when *B. infantis* eats HMOs, it releases sialic acid into the gut and bloodstream—a nutrient required for brain development and cognition. So all those complex sugars that are so abundant in human milk but lacking in the milk of other animals, may play a profound role in the development of our brains, thanks to the bacteria in our gut.

Where does *B. infantis* come from? Somehow, in ways we don't yet fully understand, the body recruits these bacteria into the milk ducts so they can colonize the mother's milk. Yes, human milk is not sterile. There's even evidence that the microbial populations of breast milk are not limited to *B. infantis*. It could be that milk is a probiotic as well as providing all the right nutrients. But we need a lot more research on this before we are able to make full sense of this finding.

Meanwhile, HMOs have another nifty function. They fight off pathogens by acting as decoys. When viruses and bacteria invade your baby's gut, the HMOs directly prevent them from sticking to mucosal surfaces.

The sialic acid that *B. infantis* produces can also be found in breast milk and appears to help with infant development. In the

African nation of Malawi, almost half of all children under age five show stunted growth even though they are exclusively breast-fed early in life. Other breast-fed babies, from similar households and backgrounds, grow normally. To find out why, researchers collected milk samples from mothers whose babies were stunted or normal and compared their composition.[4] The breast milk of mothers with healthy babies was richer in sugars containing sialic acid, a compound that supports rapid brain development in infants.

Since gut microbes are important mediators of normal growth and development, scientists looked to an animal model to explore the relative roles of diet and microbes. First, they fed bacteria from the feces of an undernourished infant to mice or piglets. Then they fed the animals a typical Malawian diet of corn, legumes, vegetables, and fruit, which on its own does not promote healthy growth. In this model, the animals resembled undernourished Malawian babies transitioning to solid foods.

Next, the researchers isolated sialic acid from cow's milk. When they added it to the insufficient diet, the animals flourished. They gained weight, grew bigger bones, and showed metabolic changes in their livers, muscles, and brains, indicating an ability to mobilize more nutrients from their food. But these effects depended almost entirely on the presence of gut microbes.

By isolating and growing the donated gut bacteria in a dish, the scientists were able to tease out which strains were affected by the sialylated sugars. They saw that one species fed on the sugars whereas another fed on the digested products of those sugars. So the sialic acid was feeding a microbial factory that in some way influenced growth. So far researchers have not figured out how these microbes influence growth, but as we always say, this is an area of active research.

What if I can't breast-feed?

We often get questions about possible differences between breast milk and formula. Is breast milk "better" because of what it contains or is there something bad or missing in formula? Is it important to keep your baby away from all formula, even at the expense of having them go a little hungry? Is a little breast milk enough to help give your baby an early advantage?

Questions like these went from abstract discussions of theoretical interest to immense practical importance for Rob and Amanda days after their daughter was born.

The first week with their new baby was rocky—she cried a lot and seemed uninterested in nursing. Frazzled and frightened, they visited a lactation specialist, who weighed the child on an extremely sensitive scale before and after a feeding. The difference was only a few grams. As gently as she could, the specialist informed Amanda, "Your baby is crying because she's hungry. You're not producing enough milk." Then their baby wasn't the only one crying: there are few worse nightmares for a new mother than being unable to adequately nourish her child.

This led Rob and Amanda to a quest through the scientific literature on what was best for their baby. It was easy to find studies promoting the idea that breast milk is good. But what if you *can't* make enough milk? There are also lots of studies showing that early malnutrition is one of the worst things that can happen to a baby, leading to many kinds of health problems, including cognitive ones. Babies who do not get enough to eat early on can become both sickly and retarded. They face a higher heart attack risk and are less able to hold down a job later in life (presumably due to cognitive effects).

The worried couple consulted a parade of doulas, lactation consultants, nurses, psychiatrists, and other specialists for advice, but Amanda's milk production stubbornly refused to increase. What was plan B to keep their baby fed? Should they supplement with formula, or would exposing their baby to its "artificial ingredients" lead to even worse outcomes? Can formula be augmented to resemble breast milk? Should they use human milk from another woman?

Since they wanted to stay as close to mother's milks as possible, they decided to try pasteurized human milk from the milk bank in Denver. After braving rush hour traffic to make the sixty-mile round trip, Rob proudly obtained a few four-ounce bottles of human milk. Their daughter drank greedily, burped happily, and settled down to sleep. But the milk didn't last long. They were back the next day. And the next. Soon they were spending over $1,000 a week on milk as their baby's voracious appetite increased. She was finally getting access to the nutrition she had craved all along, but the escalating costs were unsustainable.

At that point, they started to wonder: is there any evidence that *pasteurized* human milk is more beneficial than formula? Pasteurization heats milk to kill dangerous bacteria. That also kills off good bacteria and destroys beneficial chemicals and antibodies that mothers naturally pass on to their babies in breast milk. Also, while there is substantial evidence that breast-fed babies do better than bottle-fed ones in many areas of health, it's not clear that pasteurized milk from a donor mother whose baby is older or younger than yours will do the same. A mother's milk changes as her infant matures but, as far as we know, milk banks don't try to match donors and recipient babies by age. Unfortunately, tests directly comparing regular breast milk to pasteurized breast milk to formula have not been done, leaving parents facing nursing difficulties to find their own way.

Rob and Amanda weighed the few knowns and many unknowns, and switched to a different approach: they stopped the milk-bank deliveries and instead gave their daughter all the un-pasteurized, microbe-building milk Amanda could pump, while making up the difference in their baby's appetite with formula. With the money they saved, they hired night nurses so they could both get a good night's sleep from time to time—which has been shown to help increase milk production as well as decreasing post-partum depression.

What they learned was that when deciding to address a particular issue regarding your baby's microbiome, you want to consider whether you're spending your time and resources effectively to address the bigger issues. Because let's face it, you won't be able to address everything.

So don't worry too much if you're not able to breast-feed: the differences relative to some of the advanced formulas coming on the market today are probably small. Although your child may not be getting your personal probiotics or antibodies, you're definitely better off making sure that your baby gets enough to eat.

Is formula safe?

Yes, formula is safe, but it's not a perfect substitute for breast milk. New mothers choose to formula-feed for many reasons. They cannot produce enough milk, or find breast-feeding extremely painful, or have recurring infections (mastitis). Some women have work schedules that make frequent feedings difficult, or they want their spouses or partners to help out during the night, but they detest using breast pumps to store up extra milk for these situations. Others must take medications that would be harmful to their baby if transmitted in the breast milk. In short, there are lots of reasons why breast-feeding won't work for everyone.

For decades, infant formula was based almost entirely on cow's milk because it is by far the most widely available kind of milk. However, the balance of nutrients between cow's milk and human milk is different. Both the macronutrients (protein, fats, and carbohydrates) and the micronutrients (vitamins, minerals, and so on) are not equivalent, reflecting the specific nutritional needs and growth patterns of the different species, both mammalian and microbial. Additionally, some of the proteins in cow's milk can be difficult for some children to digest. Infant formula is therefore modified to adjust the balance of macronutrients, fortified with additional micronutrients, and the protein is hydrolyzed (broken up into smaller pieces in "gentle" formulas for fussier infants) to reduce the difficulty in digestion and the risk of allergies.

As discussed in the section on breast milk, recent studies have revealed that it contains a spectacular ingredient—human milk oligosaccharides, or HMOs.[5] They are complex sugars that feed the microbes in your baby's gut. And these HMOs are entirely different from oligosaccharides in cow's milk.

Realizing the importance of HMOs, formula manufacturers are looking for ways to improve their products. But there's a rub. HMOs are only made by humans. Oligosaccharides in the milk of farm animals are much less abundant and structurally less complex. They are not a substitute. Plus no one has yet found a way to extract exact analogues of HMO from other natural sources or to modify the oligosaccharides from other species to match HMOs. Consequently, the best they can do is to add to the formula oligosaccharides from chicory, yeast, and bacteria that weakly mimic HMOs.

Given evidence that intact cow's milk protein raises the risk for common allergic and autoimmune diseases—such as asthma, eczema, food allergies, and type 1 diabetes—formula manufacturers nowadays sell hydrolyzed cow's milk. Infant feeding guidelines in the United States, Europe, and Australasia recommend these formulas in the hope that they may prevent infant and childhood allergies, and are unlikely to do any harm.

Newer formulas are also enriched with prebiotics (fertilizer for the bacteria, including but not limited to HMOs), probiotics (such as *Bifidobacterium* and *Lactobacillus*), and synbiotics (a combination of both). These newer formulas are thought to be effective in reducing a range of conditions, including colic and asthma.

But a study published in March 2016 casts serious doubt on the ability of these formulas to prevent allergies.[6] In a systematic review and meta-analysis of thirty-seven trials involving nineteen thousand participants carried out between 1946 and 2015, researchers found no consistent evidence to support current recommendations. And claims that hydrolyzed formulas protect against allergies might lead some women to abandon breast-feeding by convincing them incorrectly that the products are superior to their own milk.

But to reiterate: if you choose to not breast-feed or find that you cannot, you don't need to feel guilty. Although many studies show some advantages of breast-feeding, the most likely outcome for a formula-fed child is that the child will be perfectly healthy. Some of the best-controlled studies have shown smaller advantages to breast-feeding when confounding factors like socioeconomic status are taken into account. However, all major health agencies, including the AAP, do recommend breast-feeding where possible for a variety of well-researched reasons relating to both infant and maternal health.

Is milk from a wet nurse or milk bank safe?

Milk from a milk bank is pasteurized, so it's safe from the perspective of not containing any known pathogens. But it also loses any benefits from live microbes, proteins (including antibodies) that can be unfolded during the pasteurization process, or small molecules like some kinds of oligosaccharides that break down easily with heating.

At commercial milk banks, rigorous screening and controls are in place to prevent microbial contamination in processing.[7] However, if you buy milk from mothers who sell it as a sideline, you might be risking potential infections, or even a wide range of drugs, both legal and illegal, that are passed from mother to breast milk. Milk from a wet nurse can contain harmful microbes, notably HIV, medications such as antibiotics and antidepressants, and environmental toxins such as phthalates and mercury. All these can be transmitted in breast milk, so you want to choose your wet nurse with your baby's health in mind.

And you might want to know where she's from. For example, in countries where women eat fish containing high levels of mercury, human breast milk can be toxic. Additionally, if your wet nurse has infected and inflamed nipples or mastitis, the bacteria causing that infection can hurt your baby. On the other hand, human milk is the best food for your infant. Our advice: use common sense when choosing a supplier.

Do dietary supplements pass through breast milk?

Sometimes. The good news is that if you're healthy and eat well, dietary supplements are not likely to influence nutrient levels in your breast milk.[8] This was demonstrated in a study of Italian mothers who ate a traditional Italian diet (meaning it was well-balanced) while breast-feeding their full-term babies.[9] The moms were divided into two groups. One took a supplement containing zinc, copper, and potassium iodide—trace elements recommended for nursing mothers. The second did not take the supplement. After three months, no differences were seen in the two groups in terms of the quality of their milk or health of their infants. The supplements did not matter.

Similarly, a study of nursing mothers in The Gambia, Africa, found that dietary supplements had little influence on the volume of milk produced, despite the fact that the women on dietary supplements ate more calories.[10]

On the other hand, the active ingredient in fatty fish such as salmon, tuna, and mackerel—a compound called DHA, or docosahexaenoic acid—does pass from your diet into your breast milk in a dose-dependent manner.[11] The more food containing DHA that you eat, the more your baby gets. DHA is a vital component for the growth and functional development of infant brains. Babies fed formula without DHA later developed a number of health problems, including depression and attention deficit disorder. Fortunately, DHA is a natural component of breast milk, and is now added to infant formula.

Fish oil is also good for nursing mothers. It alters breast milk fatty acids in a good way and promotes positive immune function in their infant's gut lining by increasing the abundance of microbes that make short-chain fatty acids.[12]

If you're lactating, your body knows how to make milk. It may be possible to slightly alter that milk through diet, but you cannot fundamentally change it. However, if you can't produce enough breast milk on your own, dietary supplements will not help you. Though Irish mothers swear by unpasteurized Guinness, which is full of microbial brewer's yeast, you'd have to live in Ireland to get hold of it.

Do antibiotics pass through my breast milk? If so, how might this affect my baby's microbiome?

Breast milk is without a doubt the best nutritional source for your baby. But sometimes you may need to take an antibiotic to treat an infection while you are breast-feeding. Antibiotics can pass into breast milk and from there into your baby, and while their administration during breast-feeding is accepted as necessary, it is important to understand some of the potential risks.

Obviously, if you need the antibiotic you should take it. If you're not sure, please have a frank discussion with your doctor about the potential consequences of taking it or not. Most doctors are well aware of the risks and will provide a balanced perspective. At the same time, because many patients demand antibiotics even for ailments that won't benefit from them, such as viral infections, some doctors are likely to give you a prescription because they're worried that you won't leave happy without one. So it may help to reassure them that you're not that kind of patient.

If you must take the drug, you can find ways to avoid exposing your baby. One is to locate a breast milk bank (although, as Rob and Amanda found, this route can be very expensive, in part because of the rigorous screening that milk banks do to guard against pathogens). Make sure that the bank you are working with screens their donors for antibiotic use.

If antibiotic-free breast milk is not an option, then you need to know some things. First, not all mothers are alike. The degree to which an antibiotic will be transferred from your blood into your breast milk is highly variable; each mother has a different rate of absorption, but the factors that determine this are poorly understood.[13]

Second, the length of each feeding can matter. Twenty years

ago, lactation specialists differentiated between foremilk and hindmilk. But don't be confused. These are not two types of milk. Hindmilk simply arrives a bit later than foremilk and is higher in fat and alkalinity. The issue here is that hindmilk is likely to have a higher concentration of the antibiotic, so the longer infants suckle, the more likely they are to get a dose of the drug.

Third, the type of antibiotic is important.[14] Breast tissue can metabolize sulfa drugs, such as Bactrim and Sulfazine, rendering them less effective. Sulfa drugs are an older class of antimicrobial agents still in use, although they can produce a variety of unpleasant side effects. It has not been established how breast tissue causes these drugs to lose their activity, but it's likely that their ability to act as antibiotics is altered in some way; it is also possible that microbes chemically modify them here as they do in other parts of the body. Other types of antibiotics do not appear to be affected by breast tissue.

Finally, as we noted above, your baby's age may make a big difference. An infant's microbiome undergoes huge fluctuations during early phases of life, and the chemical composition of the breast milk (and possibly the input of microbes in the breast milk itself) also changes over time. Given these changes, an antibiotic could retard or delay the microbiome from bouncing back and recovering or developing normally. However, please be aware that "normal" microbiome development is still not a concept that is fully understood.

In both adults and infants, antibiotics cause a significant decrease in the abundance of major bacterial species in the gut, suppressing the existing microbiome. This removes a primary barrier against disease-causing organisms, which could make your baby more susceptible to gut infections and possibly other systemic infections. Changes in the gut microbiome can also lead to shifts in gut chemistry (especially due to the changes in bile acid metabolism), leading to inflammation and diarrhea. Suppression of the gut microbiome, especially certain species of *Enterobacter*, can also lead to a proliferation of yeasts such as *Candida*. The result is often thrushlike symptoms, especially noticeable around the rectum. (Dylan, Jack's son, had this several times during infancy.)

A number of antibiotics have been designated as safe for use during breast-feeding (aminoglycosides, amoxicillin, amoxicillin-clavulanate, antitubercular drugs, cephalosporins, macrolides, trimethoprim-sulfamethoxazole). All others should be treated with caution or not used. However, even these "safe" antibiotics can cause shifts in the gut microbiome, which could have unknown consequences. And safety testing at the FDA never takes the microbiome into account—or at least not yet.

The best option is to avoid breast-feeding if you have to take an antibiotic. But if you cannot avoid it, one of the antibiotics designated as safe above may be the best option, based on existing research on health outcomes for children whose mothers have taken these antibiotics.

What causes colic? Are microbes to blame?

About one in five newborns will develop symptoms of colic starting around two weeks of age. Your baby will cry inconsolably for three hours at a time—or more. Her tummy may harden and her legs stiffen between shrieks. Her face turns red. You cannot soothe her. It is agonizing.

Are microbes involved in this excruciating condition? A recent review found that colicky infants were colonized with significantly higher levels of Proteobacteria and had fewer kinds of microbes than unaffected infants.[15] Proteobacteria include species known to produce gas as well as inflammation, which may cause pain in an immature gut. In another study, babies who had fewer kinds of several well-known beneficial microbes cried more and were fussier.[16] But we don't yet know if such differences are a cause or an effect of colic. It might be that having colic changes the microbiome.

Nevertheless, probiotics may help colicky babies. Babies who got five drops of *Lactobacillus reuteri* daily in an oil suspension for three months had fewer gastrointestinal upsets such as colic, reflux, and constipation than infants who got drops that looked and tasted just the same but didn't have the probiotic.[17] The study was large (238 treated and 230 placebo) and double-blinded, meaning that neither the parents and nor the researchers knew the content of the drops in advance. These types of blinded studies are important because they mean that the researchers and the parents don't inadvertently change the results or their perceptions of how the baby is doing based on whether they're getting the probiotics.

6

....

Antibiotics

Are antibiotics absolutely necessary if my baby was exposed to meconium?

Not necessarily. When Jack's son Dylan was born in a hospital, there was some confusion during the birthing process about when Katharine could push. The attending nurse suggested that although everything seemed fine, she would need to have a doctor come and give the okay—and the doctor was held up with another delivery. This led to Jack and Katharine having to wait for a prolonged period of time, during which Dylan's head was being forced up against the pelvic bone by the increasing contractions. Obviously, this was not a comfortable experience for Katharine, but for Dylan it must have been quite traumatic. He suffered a hematoma (a swelling on his head underneath the skin) and also voided his bowel in the birth canal. This first stool, called meconium, is composed of intestinal epithelial cells, mucus, amniotic fluid, bile, and water. Unlike feces that come later, it is tarlike and usually dark olive green because of the bile acids. When infants release meconium in the birth canal, they may be delivered with telltale stained amniotic fluid. This event occurs in up to 22 percent of term births, especially in "late babies" born past the fortieth week. Dylan was born exactly at term. He has always been a very prompt child.

The risk of meconium is poorly understood, but obstetricians worry that some of these newborns could inhale the meconium-stained fluid into their lungs.[1] When this occurs, about 5 percent of such babies will develop so-called meconium aspiration syndrome. It's usually harmless, but in rare cases it can lead to death from some sort of bacterial infection.

But the phenomenon is confusing. Most research suggests that the fetus is sterile while encased in the amniotic sack and so is the meconium. Therefore, amniotic fluid tainted with meconium is unlikely to be the source of an infection. Of course it's possible that some unknown component of meconium could cause an inflammatory response in the body, potentially leaving the baby (and somehow the mother) more susceptible to infection.[2] But we don't know what it might be.

In the name of abundant caution, the standard hospital procedure for babies born with meconium in their amniotic fluid is a course of antibiotics. When Dylan was prescribed the drug, Jack and Katherine did not argue. This was their first child and they just assumed that the doctors and nurses knew best. However, very little is known about how the prophylactic use of antibiotics might influence the health of either mother or child. Only one such study was performed to a high standard, meaning that the results could be trusted, and it found no improvement in outcomes after the use of antibiotics. This suggests that Dylan did not need the drug just because he voided his colon during birth. And it led his parents to wonder how such treatment might have impacted Dylan's burgeoning microbiome.

Can I refuse antibiotics when having a vaginal birth?

The ultimate decision about what treatments to take or decline should be up to you, the patient. However, if you have a medical condition that requires antibiotics, or a vaginal pathogen that you could transmit to your baby, like group B streptococcus or gonorrhea, the risk to your baby greatly outweighs the theoretically small benefits of avoiding antibiotics early in life.

It's also not clear how much the antibiotics you take right before birth will affect your newborn. In general, share your concern with your doctor about whether antibiotics are necessary, and ask what would be the consequences of not taking them. Many physicians still espouse the belief that antibiotics can't hurt and might help. We now know that is not true.

Should my newborn get antibiotic eyedrops?

This is complicated. Among developed countries, the prophylactic administration of antibiotic eyedrops in newborns is now only found in the United States.[3] In fact, when Jack was first asked about it after a seminar he gave in Philadelphia, he didn't know what to say. He had never heard of the practice. It's not done in the United Kingdom, where his children were born. But here it is well-established—so much so that in New York State parents are not allowed to refuse the drops. If they do, the hospital has the right to call child services for failure to comply. Similarly, when confronted with the antibiotic eyedrops at the birth of their daughter in Colorado, Rob and Amanda didn't really know what to say and were strongly urged to accept them (which they did). However, on finding out afterward that they were only necessary for diseases they were sure they did not have, and when the baby had been delivered by unplanned C-section anyway, they were not happy to find out that the treatment had been unnecessary.

To understand why this treatment is used, we have to go back to the late nineteenth century, when there were high rates of ophthalmia neonatorum—neonatal conjunctivitis, or more commonly, pinkeye. In Europe, 10 percent of newborn children were developing pinkeye, and 3 percent of them went blind. One doctor, Carl Credé, noticed that this form of pinkeye only occurred in children born vaginally to mothers who had gonorrhea. He went on to prove that the pinkeye was actually caused by the gonorrhea bacterium, *Neisseria gonorrhoeae*, and decided to treat all infants born vaginally with silver nitrate eyedrops. This almost completely eradicated the disease. But it turns out that silver nitrate is nasty. It can cause chemical burns and temporary blindness itself.

Soon after this finding became public knowledge, other researchers found that infant pinkeye was caused by both gonorrhea and chlamydia. These bacterial conditions remain the only two known causes of the disease. Both are sexually transmitted and were much more common in the late nineteenth century than they are now. However, because of our diverse population, American health authorities decided that prophylactic use of an antibiotic ointment or eyedrop should be given to all newborns within an hour of their birth—just in case. The logic was, basically, "Well, why not? Antibiotics are safe and don't have any nasty side effects. Let's just do it."

Fast-forward to today. It turns out that some of the antibiotics in use don't even work on both diseases. So if a woman is screened for these pathogens, as nearly all pregnant women are in the United States, and they are shown to be negative, then why are their babies still given antibiotic eyedrops? It is possible that they could have contracted the disease after screening but before birth, although such a scenario is rare.

One obvious reason why the use of such eyedrops is a bad idea concerns antibiotic resistance. Could this ubiquitous practice be leading to an increase in resistant bacteria found in the eye? In short, we don't know. It has not been investigated effectively. But we would be very surprised if this were not the case.

The other obvious problem is that the eye microbiome is a first line of defense against conjunctivitis and other eye diseases. It's possible that removing or disrupting the microbiome at this early stage could increase an infant's susceptibility to eye infections. Again, surprisingly, there are no studies to determine if this is the case.

What exactly can antibiotics do to my gut and to my baby's gut?

A: What antibiotics do to your baby's gut depends both on your baby and on the antibiotic. If two babies have the same species of bacteria in their gut (say, *E. coli*), and they both take the same antibiotic, sometimes that antibiotic will kill that species in one of them but not the other. Scientists are still trying to find out why. It might be because of other bacteria in the gut that stop the antibiotic from working properly or absorb it preferentially, or it might be because the same species of bacteria can be more susceptible to the antibiotic at different stages in its growth. In any case, there's still a lot we don't know about why antibiotics work better for some people and some bacteria than for others, although the general prescription guidelines for antibiotics have certainly saved a lot of lives.

In general, different antibiotics target different kinds of bacteria. However, a single bacterial species can comprise both good and bad organisms (much like humans). For example, some forms of *E. coli* are harmful while others, like *E. coli* Nissle, are beneficial and are even sold as probiotics (though not in the United States, where the FDA classes it as a medicine). When you take an antibiotic, you tend to wipe out a lot of good bacteria while trying to get at the bad ones. It's like weeding with a bulldozer instead of a trowel. In addition, after a course of antibiotics, bad bacteria may grow back more quickly than good ones, like weeds sprouting up after a forest fire.

The same principles apply to other drastic therapies targeting microbes. When Rob's daughter developed recurring skin infections, the infectious disease specialist they saw suggested decolonization, which was basically a series of harsh chemical baths. When Rob dug into the scientific literature, he saw that although the procedure worked in the short term, it tended to leave the baby vulnerable to reinfection after a few months, either with the same bacteria or with other bacteria. So they decided not to do it, since the infections weren't life threatening or antibiotic-resistant.

In general, after antibiotics, the microbial community is substantially reduced in diversity. Bad bacteria like harmful strains of *E. coli* and even really bad bacteria like *Clostridium difficile* and *Staphylococcus aureus* can take over (although, fortunately, usually briefly).[4] We see more inflammation in the gut and body because of chemicals that are produced by the bad bacteria and that are recognized by the immune system, which activates an inflammatory response.

A big problem with antibiotics is that they wipe out good bacteria that make many beneficial compounds such as short-chain fatty acids (which feed the immune cells lining your gut and help control inflammation), amino acids, and vitamins. All of these decrease in number. The bacteria left behind after antibiotics don't have the productivity of the more complete ecosystem.

So although antibiotics are lifesaving when they're needed, it's a good idea to minimize their use when they're not needed. It's always worth asking your doctor what the consequences of not taking antibiotics would be and whether you can wait it out. Meanwhile, watch your baby's health closely and if the situation gets worse, start the antibiotics.

Can antibiotics in the first six months of a baby's life lead to obesity?

Quite possibly. Ever wonder how farm animals are fattened up? Back in the 1940s farmers discovered that cows, chickens, sheep, and pigs fed antibiotics gained weight and muscle mass more quickly that animals fed a drug-free diet. They quickly realized that "subtherapeutic" doses of antibiotics (that is, doses lower than the amount that would be used to treat an infection) promote growth, packing an extra 5, 10, or 15 percent of body weight onto each animal. They also learned that timing is important. For growth promotion—the ability to convert food calories into body mass—the best time to feed antibiotics is when the animals are young. Older animals do not respond as well. And animals that are germ-free, meaning they have been bred in isolation from the microbial world, and so lack any bacteria anywhere on or in their body, do not react at all to the antibiotic therapy. For the weight gain to happen, you need microbes.

Now let's look at how this picture applies to humans. It takes time for a baby's microbiome to stabilize. It's incredibly dynamic and does not acquire adult-like features until about age three.

Many things can disrupt or influence this ongoing process, including major dietary shifts, infections, environmental exposures—and antibiotics. As you know, antibiotics are designed to kill pathogens. The earliest antibiotics were narrow-spectrum, meaning they were meant to attack just one type of bug. Later, drug companies formulated broad-spectrum antibiotics to wipe out a wide variety of microbes—a kind of scorched-earth approach.

Now let's suppose your doctor prescribed a broad-spectrum antibiotic for your baby's ear infection. When the drug reaches the swollen eardrum, it knocks back the infection and may reduce inflammation and lessen the pain. But think about where else the drug goes. When it reaches your baby's gut, which is healthy and busily self-organizing, it can pack a whammy. Many species of good bacteria will get knocked back for days to weeks before rebounding. Some rare species may even be exterminated. In fact, in studies of adults given antibiotics repeatedly, their microbiomes are still different months to years later and may never recover.[5] This discussion applies mainly to oral and intravenous antibiotics, and topical antibiotics in general have less effect on the rest of the body.

Lots of children are being affected by antibiotics. The average American child has received nearly three antibiotic courses by age two, about ten courses by age ten, and around seventeen courses by age twenty. This is remarkable: at a course of antibiotics per year on average, we'd expect to see big changes in the microbiome from the repeated disturbance to the ecosystem.

So what are the consequences of early exposure to antibiotics? We know that gut bacteria help modulate your baby's metabolism. A variety of microbes consume the food your baby eats, extracting energy that is then passed along to their growing body. Interestingly, bacteria can also influence the way your baby's body processes energy, although exactly how they do this is not well understood. We know that bacterial metabolites—and changes to the immune system wrought by the presence of certain bacteria—can alter how your baby's liver functions, which can in turn affect how much fat his or her body lays down. They can also affect other aspects of your baby's metabolism, possibly leading to obesity and even diabetes. (This has been well established in animal models, mostly mice, and although the relevance to human disease is plausible, the picture is somewhat less clear.)

Therefore, not surprisingly, the result of early exposure to antibiotics is that kids get fatter.[6] According to Dr. Martin Blaser, director of NYU's Human Microbiome Program, "Giving our children antibiotics may be a factor in fueling the rise in obesity as well as other diseases that have emerged since World War II. Clearly antibiotics are necessary some of the time, but we need to learn how to use them more judiciously." A study of over twenty-eight thousand mother-child pairs from the Danish National Birth Cohort found that antibiotic exposure in children during the first six months of life was associated with an increased risk of being overweight at age seven.[7] However, another study involving 38,522 kids and 92 pairs of twins found that exposure to antibiotics did not produce statistically significant evidence of weight gain.[8] So the results are conflicting, and there must be more to it.

Paradoxically, high levels of antibiotics in early childhood can also stunt your baby's growth. In studies using mice, the same kinds of antibiotics that caused some animals to gain weight also caused others to lose weight.[9] This variation was driven in part by the size of the antibiotic dose, the strain of mouse used, and the diet of the mouse. Fortunately, in humans, the risk for obesity is relatively small compared to many other factors, such as diet. (This is true in mice as well.) We know, for example, that a high-fat, high-sugar diet has a much greater probability of leading to obesity than the number of doses of antibiotics a child has taken. A similar trend is also seen for sedentary behavior—kids who are more active are less likely to become obese, and being inactive is a much greater predictor of obesity than whether the child took antibiotics. However, there is some controversy over whether activity prevents obesity or whether the metabolic changes that lead to obesity also make people less active.

7

Probiotics

What are probiotics good for?

It depends on the probiotic. On the one hand, probiotics have been around for centuries. They form part of our ancestral and contemporary diets and have long been associated with positive health benefits. The World Health Organization defines probiotics as "live microorganisms which, when administered in adequate amounts, confer a health benefit on the host." They are found in many foods, including yogurt, kefir, sauerkraut, and other fermented products. They are also found in breast milk.

On the other hand, most commercially available probiotics make torrents of health claims that simply have not been supported by research. A pill with "40 billion live organisms" is not going to help your child lose weight or "boost" their immune system. It won't stop your baby from crying on an airplane, protect your toddler's teeth from decay, lessen the duration of a cold or flu, or cure acid reflux. It's a billion-dollar industry with virtually no medical oversight.

One question we almost always get: should my child eat yogurt? Well, basically there's is no credible evidence that the regular consumption of a probiotic yogurt (whether dairy or non-dairy) will make your child or you any healthier. But this doesn't stop marketers from suggesting that it's a delicious panacea. Jack eats yogurt regularly, mainly because he likes it. He encourages his children to eat it. Yogurt with live active cultures is a probiotic in that it can have health benefits, but only very specific health benefits—which we will get to these later. Yogurt contains living bacteria, such as *Lactobacillus delbrueckii* and *Streptococcus thermophilus*. It may also contain other strains of *Lactobacillus* and *Bifidobacteria*. Food manufacturers may not like to admit it, but it is difficult to control the types of organisms that grow in these live cultures, despite industry standards set to determine what types of bacteria should be in yogurt. Rob also eats a lot of live yogurt, especially Icelandic skyr, but more for the flavor than for specific microbial health benefits. Jack eats a lot of sheep-milk yogurt, which is naturally lactose-free, but again mainly because of the taste.

As far back as the late nineteenth century, Nobel laureate Elie Metchnikoff was suggesting that regular consumption of fermented cow's milk could enhance overall health and even delay the onset of age-related neurological decline. Admittedly, Elie did predict many of the basic tenets of our understanding of the microbiome and human physiology that we accept today. But despite more than a hundred years of research we have still to find credible support that his theories about regular consumption of probiotics were correct.

Many types of probiotics are sold for all sorts of conditions, but very few of them have been vetted in published literature, with appropriately designed trials that would allow us to evaluate whether they actually work. It might not be advisable to give a probiotic to your child unless you need to—and even then you should select one that has been shown to help kids with the condition you are dealing with. Otherwise you're likely to throw away your money.

On the other hand, you probably can't avoid encountering them in the supplement aisles of your local pharmacy or grocery story. Over the last twenty to thirty years there has been an explosion in the development of bacterial cultures that are sold as liquids or in the form of pills full of preserved spores. So are these new probiotics any better?

The answer is, we still don't know. The lack of clinical trials demonstrating efficacy is the major obstacle to knowing whether they are better than existing formulations that have been shown clinically to help with diarrhea and atopy. On the other hand, manufacturers of some newer probiotics are beginning to build a case for their products. For example, VSL#3 is a mixture of eight diverse bacterial strains that has been shown to benefit kids with irritable bowel syndrome or ulcerative colitis and adults after surgical removal of their large intestine.[1] VSL#3 influences the immune system mostly by inducing anti-inflammatory pathways. In fact, Jack tried VSL#3 to reduce joint pain and found it quite effective. However, the claims that probiotic mixtures will help to support overall health are still woefully unproven.

The idea behind probiotics is seductive. It's called dysbiosis. The term simply means a microbial imbalance on or inside the body. It has many causes—overuse of antibiotics, lousy diet, contaminated food or water, disease, and so on.

Gut microbes live together harmoniously. They check each other's growth, produce food, vitamins, amino acids, and other beneficial compounds for your child's body to use. They both stimulate and control your child's immune system and hormonal balance, and even their neurons. But when gut microbes fall out of balance, the community becomes disturbed. This collapse of equilibrium has unpredictable consequences. Some bacteria can overgrow, others starve and disappear, and some will just shut up shop and wait it out, entering a type of dormancy, like a seed waiting for the right conditions to germinate.

Probiotics are useful when your child's gut, skin, or other tissues experience dysbiosis. They contain friendly bacteria, many of which are analogous to the bacteria that normally live in the gut, and they can bring balance back to the equation. When the equilibrium of your child's microbiome is disrupted—when they have dysbiosis—probiotics may help rescue the community, resetting it to their personal norm.

We expect this, though we actually have limited evidence to support the assumption, and we still don't really understand why it could occur. One theory is that the mass of cells in a probiotic drink or yogurt can activate immune responses that reduce inflammation or alter the way the immune system interacts with the microbiome.[2] Think of the immune system as a gardener, keeping the bacteria it wants healthy and active and removing the ones that it doesn't want around. The immune system during dysbiosis is more like a drunk gardener, making very bad choices. A probiotic seems to act to rebalance the immune system and therefore indirectly rebalance the microbiome.

We have no evidence that probiotics really hang around in your child's gut. Many commonly available probiotics seem to mostly be excreted, so the only way they could possibly change the body is by interacting with the immune system. Or perhaps they compete for nutrients (albeit briefly) with their existing microbes before being summarily ejected. It's possible that taking a probiotic early in life—before the microbiome has stabilized to an adult form—could lead to some bacteria becoming part of an infant's microbiome. But that would not be the sort of probiotic you can buy in the drugstore. It would be the next generation of probiotics we are currently developing. These are based around bacteria that are isolated from humans and selected to fulfill a specific health-promoting role in the developing gut.

Despite the lack of evidence that regular consumption of probiotics provides specific health benefits, many people will tell you they think their children are healthier because of them. Are they acting as a placebo? The answer can be complicated to pin down. Ideally we should be able to measure improvement in some specific aspect of health. But the benefits can also include things that are simply felt or perceived, without being measurable. We have much to learn.

So when should you give a probiotic to your child? If you are currently breast-feeding, then you are already doing so. There is a wealth of evidence to suggest that if your child has diarrhea, it can be treated with a probiotic. If your child has had an operation, many pediatric surgeons will recommend Greek yogurt for its nutritional and probiotic benefit, especially to reduce the likelihood of bacterial overgrowth in the intestine. Here are a few examples of other times you can give your child a probiotic.

Food Allergies

Probiotics can treat food allergies, which, over the past decade, have risen by as much as 20 percent in developed societies.

Cow's milk allergy is one of the most common food allergies of infancy and early childhood, with an estimated prevalence of 2 to 3 percent worldwide. Symptoms include frequent spitups, vomiting, diarrhea, swollen lips or eyes, runny nose, and persistent distress. In this case, your baby cannot tolerate a protein, called casein, found in cow's milk.

Our goal is to induce tolerance by exploiting bacteria. Can probiotics help?

A small clinical trial in which Jack's laboratory participated aimed to find out.[3] Three groups of infants under three months old, all of them allergic to cow's milk, were fed formula. One received an ordinary brand. Another got formula containing an extensively hydrolyzed form of casein. In such products, the casein protein is broken down into smaller units that your baby can digest. A third group got the hydrolyzed casein plus the probiotic *Lactobacillus rhamnosus* GG.

Some of the babies who received the probiotic and hydrolyzed formula showed a significant increase in their tolerance to cow's milk. And others who got the same mixture did not.

Why not? To be honest, we are not 100 percent certain. But we found clues by looking at fecal samples of all the babies.

Those who got better had enriched strains of a type of gut bacteria that ferments carbohydrates in the colon to produce butyrate, a short chain of carbons and hydrogen atoms similar to those found in fats. Butyrate is a useful molecule. It feeds immune cells in the gut that then produce a chemical that dampens inflammation. Thus, more butyrate production in the gut means less inflammation and improved tolerance to a food allergen.

Similarly, a recent study in Australia showed that a commercial probiotic could be effective at reversing peanut allergies.[4] Thirty allergic children got a small daily dose of peanut protein together with increasing doses of the probiotic *L. rhamnosus* GG, which were eventually equivalent to eating the amount found in a whopping forty-four pounds of yogurt every day. After eighteen months, four in five kids could eat peanuts without an allergic reaction. This and other studies have recently led to a change in the AAP recommendations on peanuts, suggesting that they be introduced early rather than avoided for the first two years.

Yeast Infections, Atopic Dermatitis, and Eczema
When Jack's son Dylan had a candida infection in his bowel, the infection spread everywhere, over his skin, even his groin, for

over six months. But his mom, knowing that yogurt is often used to treat thrush infections, spread yogurt all over Dylan's skin, and both the oral and genital candida infections disappeared.

So what is going on here? Well, with a sample size of one child, we can't know for certain whether this worked for Dylan, but clinical trials have shown that yogurt, either alone or in combination with honey (full of natural antifungals and antibiotics), will work for thrush in adults and in animals. No studies have yet been done in children.

In an eczema trial, 132 mothers and their infants were given the probiotic *L. rhamnosus* GG, starting during pregnancy and continuing for six months after birth.[5] Atopic eczema was diagnosed in 46 of 132 children by the age of two. The kids who had taken probiotics were half as likely to develop eczema as the kids who didn't. The researchers followed all the kids to age four or five and found the same results. The probiotic protected the kids up to school age. Another study of pregnant women and their children got different results: 220 of the subjects got a cocktail of probiotics (*L. salivarius* CUL61, *L. paracasei* CUL08, *Bifidobacterium animalis subspecies lactis* CUL34 and *B. bifidum* CUL20) and 234 received a placebo; neither the probiotics nor the placebo appeared to affect eczema rates in the infants.[6]

A recent well-controlled study of fifty infants with eczema and fifty-one without identified different stool bacteria in the two groups.[7] At this point, the differences are just statistical associations and the changes may have nothing to do with eczema. But these kinds of studies provide us with a template for investigating possible relationships.

Ear Infections

Another study found that probiotics can reduce the number and severity of ear infections in young swimmers.[8] Forty-six girls, average age thirteen, who swam competitively were broken into two groups. One ate thirteen ounces of ordinary yogurt a day for eight weeks. The other ate a yogurt naturally enriched with live bacteria for the same amount of time. In the end, while we assume that none of the girls were particularly faster, the girls eating the probiotic yogurt experienced fewer colds and less ear pain.

In a boon to parents everywhere, probiotics have also been shown to reduce ear infections in young children.[9] Sixty-five children with a recent diagnosis of recurrent ear infections caused by the pathogen *Streptococcus pyogenes* were recruited. Forty-five were treated every day for three months with an oral, slow-release tablet containing the probiotic *S. salivarius* K12. The kids treated with K12 showed a 90 percent reduction in their episodes of sore throat and a 40 percent reduction in acute ear infections, which was significantly greater than the kids who didn't consume the probiotic.

Probiotics are an exciting medical frontier.[10] Once we know what's missing in a microbiome that is out of balance, perhaps we can restore the good stuff—and make it taste good too.

Which probiotic is best for my child?

This is one of the most difficult questions we get asked—and we are asked it a lot. Probiotics seem so easy. They are not thought of as a drug, they are natural, and they are usually available without a prescription. True, they are expensive, but the ease of use and peace of mind seems to outweigh this cost.

The first difficulty in answering the question is that we are not clinicians. We are research scientists, and as such it would be unethical for us to make an explicit recommendation. Second, most clinicians don't really know what to suggest. Table 1 includes the most up-to-date recommendations regarding probiotics and

TABLE 1. LIST OF BRANDS AND PROBIOTIC STRAINS USED TO TREAT CONDITIONS IN YOUNG CHILDREN

Brand Name	Probiotic Strain	Conditions Treated
Indication for Pediatric Health		
BioGaia ProTectis	*L. reuteri DSM 17938*	Regurgitation, gastro-intestinal motility Colic Infectious diarrhea Antibiotic-associated diarrhea Constipation Functional abdominal pain Irritable bowel syndrome Eczema
Culturelle Kids Chewables Culturelle Kids Packets	*L. rhamnosus GG*	Infectious diarrhea Antibiotic-associated diarrhea Functional abdominal pain Irritable bowel syndrome Hospital-acquired infections Eczema
Dentaq Oral and ENT Health Probiotic Complex	*S. salivarius BAA-1024* *L. plantarum SD-5870* *L. reuteri SD-5865* *L. acidolphilus SD-5212* *L. salivarius SD-5208* *L. paracasei SD-5275*	Oral health
Florastor	*Saccharomyces boulardii lyo*	Infectious diarrhea Antibiotic-associated diarrhea Clostridria-associated diarrhea prevention

(continued)

TABLE 1.

Brand Name	Probiotic Strain	Conditions Treated
		Heliobacter pylori adjunct to standard therapy
Lacidofil	*L. rhamnosus R0011* *L. helveticus R0052*	Eczema
Nestle Gerber Soothe Colic Drops	*L. reuteri 17938*	Regurgitation, gastro-intestinal motility Colic Infectious diarrhea Antibiotic-associated diarrhea Constipation Functional abdominal pain Irritable bowel syndrome Eczema
OralBiotics (BLIS K12)	*Streptococcus salivarius K12*	Oral health
Pedia-Lax Yums	*L. reuteri DSM 17938*	Regurgitation, gastro-intestinal motility Colic Infectious diarrhea Antibiotic-associated diarrhea Constipation Functional abdominal pain Irritable bowel syndrome Eczema
UP4 Junior	*B. lactis UABLA-12 4.2B*	Eczema
	L. acidophilus DDS-1 0.8B	
VSL#3	*L. acidophilus SD5212* *L. casei SD5218* *L. bulgaricus SD 5210*	Infectious diarrhea Ulcerative colitis: adjunct to standard therapy

TABLE 1.

Brand Name	Probiotic Strain	Conditions Treated
	L. plantarum SD 5209 B. longum SD 5219 B. infantis SD5220 B. breve SD 5206 S. thermophiles SD5207	Functional abdominal pain Irritable bowel syndrome
Functional Foods with Added Probiotics		
DanActive/Actimel	L. casei sp. Paracasei CNCM 1-1518	Infectious diarrhea Heliobacter pylori: adjunct to standard therapy Common infectious disease
Nestle Gerber Extensive HA Formula	B. lactis BB-12 DSM 10140	Antibiotic-acquired diarrhea Common infectious disease
Nestle Gerber Good Start Gentle for Supplementing Formula	B. lactis BB-12 DSM 10140	Antibiotic-acquired diarrhea Common infectious disease
Nestle Gerber Graduates Soothe Infant and Toddler Formula Nestle Gerber Soothe Infant Formula	L. reuteri protectis DSM 17938	Regurgitation, gastro-intestinal motility Colic Infectious diarrhea Antibiotic-acquired diarrhea

pediatric health. (For more details, see www.usprobioticguide .com.) For each disease state you can use this information to discuss with your doctor potential strategies for treating your child's illness.

Should I give my child probiotics if he has diarrhea?

Absolutely yes. This is one of the best described and best studied examples of the health-promoting benefit of probiotics. In a systematic review of a series of double-blind trials, treatment of infants with acute diarrhea using *L. rhamnosus* GG was shown to significantly reduce symptoms, severity, and duration of the condition.[11] Simply put, kids got better faster and had a less severe response when they took the probiotic. The treatment worked best with rotavirus infections—the kind that cause acute gastroenteritis.

We don't exactly understand how the probiotic induces changes that can reduce diarrhea, but it likely decreases inflammation and also competes with pathogens for nutrients and places to hang on to in the gut. Some other probiotics, including *E. coli* Nissle, have been shown to actively compete with invading pathogens that can cause diarrhea.[12] They do this by sequestering all the iron that the pathogen would normally use to fuel its growth. So if you think you might be susceptible to getting an infection, then taking this probiotic could be useful. However, while it is sold as a commercial probiotic in Europe and Canada, it is currently unavailable in the United States.

So, absolutely yes. Most clinicians should recommend a probiotic if your child has severe diarrhea.[13]

If my child has taken an antibiotic, should she also take a probiotic?

Diarrhea is a common side effect of antibiotic therapy, especially in infants. The good news is that probiotics such as *L. rhamnosus* GG can help alleviate this condition. But beware. Other probiotics have no effect; *L. rhamnosus* GG is the only one to have been clinically validated. You can buy this probiotic in virtually any major drugstore and it doesn't require a prescription. It is also part of many probiotic formulations—but always check the label. Just because it may say "contains Lactobacillus," doesn't mean it contains *L. rhamnosus* GG.

On the other hand, yogurts have been shown to help with diarrhea. Several of Rob's colleagues, including Dr. Jairam K.P. Vanamala at Penn State University, have mentioned that yogurt is a traditional remedy for diarrhea in India for both children and adults and may also act as a preventive measure.

You may be able to ward off the growth of yeasts, which can take over your child's gut after taking antibiotics, by adding probiotic bacteria to his or her diet. But we advise against probiotic yeasts (such as *Saccharomyces boulardii*) because they don't contain the bacteria needed to restore microbial balance after antibiotics.

Rob eats a lot of yogurt (carefully avoiding the kinds high in sugars or artificial sweeteners) and always encourages his daughter to eat it as well, especially on the rare occasions when she needs to take antibiotics. She especially likes it with honey, which itself has antimicrobial properties that tend to combat fast-growing "bad bacteria" like *Streptococcus* that can colonize the throat after antibiotics.

Can probiotic yogurt help cure diaper rash?

Yes. Our colleague, Dr. Rachel Jones, told us an interesting story. When her daughter had a severe diaper rash, she tried everything. She left off the diapers to let air circulate on her daughter's little bottom, which was red, raw, and hot to the touch. None of the over-the-counter creams helped. Rachel's mother told her about a traditional remedy using lightly whipped egg whites and yogurt. She was skeptical but willing to try anything. When she applied the egg white to her daughter's bottom, it appeared to cook, forming a smooth dry layer almost like a second skin. The rash improved almost immediately and was gone in thirty-six hours. When Rachel's son was born, she used a combination of egg white and yogurt to treat his thrush-associated rash. She alternated egg white and yogurt for each diaper change—and he quickly got better.

Jack has a similar story (as noted earlier). After a series of antibiotic therapies, his son Dylan had bad diarrhea and a nasty diaper rash, which essentially turned into thrush, a candida infection. As we have suggested elsewhere, a probiotic lactobacilli, such as *L rhamnosus* GG, can substantially reduce symptoms and hasten recovery from diarrhea and help suppress a yeast infection in the gut. But that's not all. You can also spread a probiotic yogurt on areas of diaper rash (around the rectum and buttocks) to alleviate a yeast infection on the skin.

In Dylan's case, his parents tried steroid creams to remove the yeast infection, but to no avail. In retrospect, this is not surprising because steroids suppress immunity, and should be used for eczema and other noninfectious skin conditions rather than infectious ones. Within days of using this yogurt treatment, however, his rash had disappeared. Obviously, we cannot generalize to all diaper rashes and all children given a few cases. Perhaps the steroid cream had a delayed response, or maybe Dylan just got better by himself. This is why we rely on larger studies with proper controls to test the efficacy of any novel treatment. Only then can we know that this or that therapy works as claimed.

What are prebiotics and what are they good for?

Prebiotics are foods, food ingredients, or additives that influence bacteria living in your child's gut. They are defined as nondigestible substances that selectively stimulate the growth and activity of one or a few types of bacteria in the colon, with the aim of improving health.

Prebiotics are typically fiber compounds, or oligosaccharides, that your child cannot digest, such as plant cell membranes made of cellulose, which make it all the way down into their lower gut or colon. There they are fermented by resident microbes, which produce other chemicals, some of which can be beneficial, such as short-chain fatty acids. Common prebiotics include galacto-oligosaccharides, oligofructose, and lactulose.[14]

If you choose to give your child a prebiotic that can be consumed by a probiotic, you may enhance the activity of the probiotic, helping it to colonize successfully.

While we are just starting to explore the potential benefits of prebiotics, it seems self-evident that feeding your child's gut microbes with the right precursors will also enhance gut metabolism. Remember, this is essentially what your baby's body does with breast milk; human milk oligosaccharides (HMOs) are produced exclusively to feed a growing microbiome. Your child's microbes produce immunological, neurological, and hormonally active metabolites that play an important role in his health. Feeding microbes the nutrients they require to produce these metabolites can only be good for your child.

The fact that most American and many European diets have abysmally low quantities of dietary fiber may help explain the explosion of immune and behavioral conditions that are so abundant in our societies. Maybe we just aren't feeding our children's microbiomes the right kind of foods! They don't produce the right chemicals and their bodies and even their brains can suffer.

What about adding dietary fiber to your child's diet. Shouldn't that help? Companies are constantly developing products such as inulin to use as a food additive. It's a naturally occurring oligosaccharide produced by many plants, usually extracted from chicory. This allows the food manufacturer to say that the food has beneficial properties because of its increased fiber content. The problem is that many of these products, including inulin, can lose some of their potency during processing. A huge body of literature deals with how these different kinds of additives lack the effects they claim. And in any case, you are likely better off increasing the amounts of whole foods containing naturally occurring prebiotics, including whole grains, legumes, leafy vegetables, and fruits such as raspberries.

Importantly, oligosaccharides are not the only prebiotics. Many other molecules can influence your child's gut microbes and improve their health. For example, curcumin, the active ingredient in turmeric, is metabolized by gut microbes to produce compounds that reduce inflammation.[15] The cancer drug cyclophosphamide, in the presence of prebiotics, can help the body mount an immune response to promote tumor suppression. And berberine, a bright yellow substance found in Oregon grape, tree turmeric, golden seal, and many other plants can alter gut microbe metabolism to reduce obesity and type 2 diabetes—but so far only in animals.[16]

In the future, we expect to be able to support the growth of specific bacteria by adding the right prebiotics, almost like fertilizer for your microbiome. Some companies are suggesting they are doing this already, but the majority of their evidence would not pass muster in the scientific literature. Clinical probiotics will be provided in concert with clinical prebiotics. This will revolutionize the impact of these products.

8

Child Diet

My baby's poop is a weird color. Is that related to changes in her microbiome or from her diet?

This is a fascinating question. We know that the composition of children's microbiome is associated with the speed at which stool transits through their body, so the consistency of their stool (as measured on the Bristol Stool Chart) correlates with changes in their microbiome.[1] But we still don't know whether their microbiome is controlling the speed of transit and consistency of their poop or if these properties indicate changes in their microbiome.

However, stool color is related to transit time. Much of the color comes from the yellowish bile acids that your child's body pumps into her gut to help with digestion. Bacteria break down these acids, affecting the color of the stool. When food moves quickly through the gut, bile acids cannot be broken down quickly, and stool color is yellowish. When food moves more slowly, the bacteria have time to break down the bile acids and process food. Your child's stool turns greenish and then, with normal movement through the digestive tract, brown.

Remember the last time you threw up? You probably saw a lot of yellow after you had cleared your stomach. That indicates a high concentration of primary bile acids. And the same is true for your baby's poop. Yellow poop is a sign of more of those undigested bile acids. Baby poop tends to be very yellow on breast milk, and somewhat browner and pastier on formula (which slows transit relative to breast milk), then changes dramatically with the introduction of solid food.

So what is a weird color? Some stool colors are concerning. White indicates an infection. Red and black indicate the presence of blood. A single stool this color may be nothing but a blip. But if you see several in a row, you should call your pediatrician.

A more serious condition, biliary atresia, which affects some four hundred newborns in the United States each year, occurs when the liver's bile ducts don't develop properly. The babies' poop is a very pale yellow or chalky gray. Recently, researchers at Johns Hopkins University developed a smartphone app, called PoopMD+, that parents can use to take photos of the contents of their babies' diapers if they suspect something is wrong.[2] Experts examine the photos and help make an initial diagnosis. Surgery to repair the bile ducts is recommended in the first month of life.

Foods can also change the color of your baby's stool. Rob's daughter's stool turned a particularly alarming shade of red after eating beets: they would have been more concerned had the coloring not affected the whole family, who were eating the same thing. Some food colorings can also pass through to your baby's stool, so if they're eating a lot of candy or drinking artificially colored beverages, that can lead to some alarming colors as well.

Should I chew food before putting it in my baby's mouth?

In many societies, mothers chew food before giving it to their babies, mainly to soften it and reduce the risk of choking. Eighty percent of babies in Nigeria receive prechewed food; in the United States one in seven caregivers overall, and more commonly African Americans, say they prechew food.

Breast milk alone will not meet your baby's nutritional needs after they turn six months old. But your child won't be able to eat adult food until about age two, when all their teeth have come in. So you face a period of blending, chopping, pureeing, or otherwise mashing up foods for them to eat. Or you can prechew.

From a microbiome perspective, we see no reason not to do this. In fact, prechewing the food may help boost your child's immune system.[3] First, premastication starts the digestive process, reducing the likelihood that food components could induce an immune reaction in your child. Many food-derived allergies are based on immune response to undigested proteins in food.[4] Second, this practice introduces complex microbes from your mouth into the food, which could help to stimulate your child's immune system responses. However, there is no scientific evidence that directly supports any immune benefit for prechewed food.

Of course, if you have some kind of oral disease, such as sore or bleeding gums, canker sores, or some other infection, then you should not be prechewing your child's food. Please use common sense.

Should I give my child dietary supplements? Children's chewable vitamins?

Many children today get a multivitamin (gummy bear or Flintstone style) along with breakfast. Parents give them as a kind of insurance policy against missing nutrients. (In fact, most adults take them for the same reason.) But if you and your child are eating healthy foods, you really don't need dietary supplements.

The first concern we often hear is whether parents should let their kids eat sugary, candy-flavored vitamins. To be honest, while refined sugar and associated sweeteners should be avoided as much as possible, the amount present in these products is extremely small, and it's not likely to have an effect.

If your child is not eating a balanced diet, then of course vitamin and mineral supplements could help to provide appropriate vitamins. Remember the slang word used to describe the English? Limeys. Why? Because the English sailors were made to consume limes on board ship to stave off vitamin C deficiency, which can cause scurvy, among other conditions. So of course if your child shows signs of diseases associated with a poor diet or malnutrition, then you need to act. But your first step should be to improve your child's diet.

An equally important question is, can excess vitamin and mineral supplements cause any harm? We know that a child's microbiome is particularly susceptible to perturbation and that, in the case of malnutrition, this can cause lasting consequences for the microbiome and for longer-term health.[5] But at this point, we simply don't know if excess supplements cause positive or negative impacts for your child's gut. There are exceptions to this general rule. For example, fat-soluble vitamins such as vitamin A are toxic at high concentrations. Polar explorers sometimes died of vitamin A poisoning after eating the livers of their dogs (the livers of carnivores have high levels of vitamin A). Vitamin D is also stored in fat and can lead to toxicity. Similarly, many minerals that are essential at low doses, such as zinc and selenium, are toxic at high doses. So you certainly shouldn't assume that if some supplements are good, more must be better, and you should consult your doctor about both the kind and amount of supplements you're using. Remember, compared to an adult, your baby is tiny. It's unwise to dose him with any substance known to be toxic in adults.

Malnourished children certainly benefit from vitamin and mineral supplements. Poor or meager diets don't provide adequate nutrients and have negative effects on the immune system, leading to increased infections of various kinds. Later in life, we see metabolic diseases linked to inflammation, including diabetes and cardiovascular disease at relatively early ages. Malnutrition also has negative effects on microbial community structure, where the microbiomes of malnourished kids are slowed in development relative to those of better-nourished children.[6] They produce less vitamins and essential amino acids, ironically increasing the dietary demand for these nutrients later on.

What solid foods are best for babies under twelve months old?

Jack's mother fed him mashed liver with honey and apparently he loved it—though it's not something he would savor today. Rob's mom swore by leafy greens and, on special occasions peas; peas are still one of his favorite vegetables, and he now likes a range of leafy greens but still hates silver beet (aka Swiss chard) even if it's fresh from the garden. Rob's daughter used to love olives when she was about a year old, but she now complains about them vociferously and picks them out of everything.

Parenting advice books are chockablock with recommendations on what to feed your baby as you transition to solid food at around six months. We tried lots of stuff, including mashed chicken, vegetables, and grains. Jack and his wife occasionally relied on processed baby foods but mostly prepared soft foods at home from fresh fruit and vegetables. This is a matter of personal preference, although we have no real understanding of the impact of the preservatives and flavor enhancers used in some commercial products on babies.

To promote a healthy microbiome in your child's gut, we recommend feeding him lots of different vegetables. Beets, carrots, corn, broccoli, and beans contain fiber, or complex indigestible carbohydrates, that can drive bacterial fermentation and produce chemicals that help regulate the immune response. Fresh fruits are also an excellent source of nutrients not found in breast milk. Apples, pears, and bananas can help to structure your baby's microbiome—and potentially help recruit new bacteria into his gut.

You can also take steps to reduce your baby's risk of developing food allergies by introducing him early on to foods that will stimulate his immune system. For example, Israeli children who ate peanut snacks were less likely to develop a peanut allergy than kids who were forbidden to eat peanuts. (See more on allergies, including the dreaded peanut allergy, in the section below.)

Your own tastes, common sense, and family food traditions can guide your choices during this transition (which, by the way, can be lots of fun). While we recommend staying away from refined sugars, a little chocolate or ice cream cannot hurt. Yogurts are good, but try to use plain yogurt instead of flavored ones— you don't want to bias your child's palate in favor of sweet foods.

The bottom line is that food preferences are learned from your family and your culture. Even one-year-old babies understand the influence of social groups in food choices. So be aware that your baby is watching what you eat and figuring out who eats what foods with whom.

What role does the microbiome play in my child's food allergies?

Food allergies are increasingly prevalent in our society. Many of you probably won't remember having friends with this problem in your preschool or elementary school years, but all that has changed. Today's classrooms are festooned with signs that say NUT-FREE ZONE and CAUTION! I HAVE FOOD ALLERGIES. DON'T FEED ME. In the last ten years, food allergies have risen by as much as 20 percent, affecting one out of every thirteen children under age eighteen. That's roughly two in every classroom.

Why are food sensitivities and food allergies increasing? First, let's look at definitions. A food allergy occurs when your baby's immune system strongly reacts to a substance (usually a protein) in a particular food shortly after it is consumed. The body misinterprets the protein as being foreign or dangerous, so it induces inflammation and releases antibodies to destroy or neutralize it. The result may be a rash, hives, nausea, stomach pain, diarrhea, shortness of breath, chest pain, a swollen tongue, or, in the worst case, swollen airways. Common food allergens are peanuts, cow's milk, tree nuts, shellfish, soy, wheat, and eggs.

A food sensitivity is a milder condition that happens up to three days after eating a particular food allergen. Your baby may be irritable or nauseated and have signs of gas, cramping, diarrhea, or heartburn. They may also suffer from hives, swelling, and itching.

The best clinical recommendation for treating food sensitivity is to avoid eating what you're allergic or sensitive to. For example, if your child reacts to cow's milk or is lactose-intolerant, don't let her drink milk or eat dairy. Of course where kids are concerned this is not always practical, as many allergens are found in complex foods, making eating out a nightmare.

But if you can manage to keep feeding the foods your child is sensitive to (at least in small amounts), there's a chance she'll become desensitized. In short, children grow out of many allergens. As many as 87 percent of kids with cow's milk allergy become desensitized within the first three years of life. Some allergists call this "spontaneous desensitization," but it's nothing of the sort. As children progress naturally toward adulthood, their microbiome shifts in ways that induce desensitization. The question is, what can we do to promote the process? How can we make it happen faster in kids where it would have happened anyway, and how can we make it happen in kids who otherwise would have remained allergic?

The role of gut microbes in food allergies and sensitivities is just coming into focus. Our bodies evolved in a sea of microbes, which found ways to communicate and cooperate. For example, some of these microbes took on the task of fermenting the fiber in our food. In so doing, they produced molecules or metabolites that help control inflammation in our guts. It's a nice example of symbiosis. We give them a home and fiber to munch; they give us a strong immune system.

But the modern world has thrown a monkey wrench into this nice picture. When your child takes too many antibiotics or you keep their world too clean, you can kill off the microbes that are tending to their immune system. Without the right microbes and their products in play, your child's immune system cannot control inflammation—and that can lead to allergies and sensitivities.

One way to ensure that your baby and toddler will be able

to control inflammation is to expose them to a diverse bacterial world. This exposure trains their immune system to identify self versus nonself, and it also increases the chance that they'll have bacteria that help keep inflammation in check.

Enter food. Peanuts and other foods contain allergens that promote inflammation. While some children may be genetically predisposed to develop a food sensitivity, most kids with food allergies just have an imbalance in their gut microbes—in other words, the wrong bugs or not enough of the right ones. On top of this, a diet high in fats and refined sugars is likely to suppress the abundance of microbes that can control inflammation. Without adequate fiber, your child's immune system may not be correctly regulated by anti-inflammatory bacteria that would normally grow on the fiber. Instead, it launches a misguided, full-blown attack against a food allergen. Sources of fiber to consider include fruit, especially bananas, salad, carrots, and other vegetables.

Your baby's gut may itself contribute to the problem. In some kids, the normal process of digesting food may be retarded or sluggish. If their microbiome is already disturbed, the food they eat may not be broken down in the right way. This slowing down could lead to a buildup of food components that could disturb their gut and induce sensitivity or an allergic response. In particular, incomplete digestion of proteins can lead to larger protein fragments that trigger an immune response, although other kinds of partially digested food can also be a problem when it gets into the large intestine.

How you prepare food can make a difference. Proteins in a liquid, soluble form are more likely to induce tolerance. Proteins in particulate form, with solid bits like roasted peanuts, are more likely to increase sensitization and induce an immune response, like hives, itchiness, or even severe swelling due to runaway inflammation. Again, this is because the solid particles are more likely to be incompletely broken down in the stomach and small intestine.

Timing is also important. Two groups of infants between four and eleven months old were assigned either to eat or not eat peanuts for up to five years.[7] Some showed a sensitivity to peanuts via a skin prick test but were not fully allergic. At the end of the study, kids who ate peanuts, including those who showed a sensitivity, were much less likely to have a peanut allergy.

In Israel, where kids eat a peanut snack called Bamba starting at a very young age, allergy rates are extremely low. The American Academy of Pediatrics recently changed its recommendations from avoiding potentially allergenic foods to introducing them early. In particular, proteins we're exposed to via our skin tend to cause allergies much more than proteins we're exposed to by eating, so it may be important to make sure that your kids eat peanut butter early rather than just smearing it all over themselves.

You are probably wondering how to stave off food allergies and sensitivities. How can you protect your baby? The prevailing strategy favored by most allergists had been to build up tolerance by injecting increasing doses of the allergen (such as milk or peanut protein) under the skin. You take your child to the allergist's office at regular intervals for shots. Yet this method had a very low success rate. According to Dr. Christina E. Ciaccio, an allergy expert and assistant professor of pediatrics at University of Chicago Medicine, "the risks of shot-based desensitization (in young children) outweigh any potential benefits and is therefore not currently used in clinical practice." A fatality in a clinical trial in the 1990s stopped it forever, she said.

Over the last ten to fifteen years, another method—oral desensitization—came into vogue, with a 50 to 75 percent success rate. This involves stimulating the children's immune response by adding the food to the mucous membranes of their mouth. Food is applied to the inside of their cheeks and onto their tongues, but the children are told to avoid swallowing so the contact with the mouth lasts longer. Although this process sounds simple, it should be done only under medical supervision: children who are highly allergic to a particular food can go into anaphylactic shock, so you don't want to take any chances.

Many researchers have tried to treat food allergies with probiotics, with wildly different results. This is not surprising given the many differences in the clinical samples, how the studies were designed, and the way the data was analyzed. But it does seem that women who take certain probiotics (*Lactobacillus acidophilus* and *Bifidobacteria*) prenatally or shortly after delivery have infants with reduced levels of an antibody produced in response to allergy.[8]

In truth, we are only starting to understand how to treat food sensitivities and allergies, but the future will likely contain a combination of oral challenge (feeding allergens early in life) and probiotic administration (like *L. rhamnosus* GG). The question remains as to whether we can treat allergies once they have already taken hold. Currently there have been no credible trials examining whether this is possible. But as we always say, this is an area of active research. We hope to get rid of all those signs in school classrooms, making food allergies and sensitivities a thing of the past.

Is it okay for my child to be a vegetarian? A vegan?

From a microbiome perspective, it's probably okay. The microbiomes of vegetarians (those who avoid meat) and vegans (those who avoid all animal products) differ significantly from those of carnivores and omnivores. But based on current research, we don't know of any nutritional aspects in meat that are required for a healthy gut (vitamin B12, often an issue on vegan diets, can be supplied in other ways such as from yeast extract). We do know that the majority of health benefits derived from your gut microbes involve the metabolism of nondigestible fibers—major components of vegetarian and vegan diets. In fact, a reduction in the abundance of bacteria that have been linked to inflammation is the major apparent health benefit of a vegan and vegetarian diet.

How diets lacking all animal protein affect growth and development in early childhood remains an active area of research. Such diets need to be very carefully monitored in order to avoid deficiency disorders.

While a vegetarian diet may seem to be healthier, it doesn't stop Jack and Rob from eating meat, mainly because it tastes good. You can feed it to your kids for the same reason. From a microbiome point of view, it won't hurt them.

So while a vegetarian diet may be perfectly healthy, eating meat, especially fish and chicken, have no known microbiome-related health issues.

What would a paleo diet look like for a kid? Would it be good for her microbiome?

The premise of a paleo diet is to avoid eating all processed foods. This means cutting out virtually everything that most of us normally feed our kids—cereal, macaroni and cheese, peanut butter and jelly, and the like. Neither Rob's nor Jack's children eat paleo diets, mostly because it is way too much trouble and we don't believe it is worth the effort.

Rob also works with the microbiomes of various people who live very traditional lifestyles, such as the Yanomami and Matsés people of the Amazon and the Hadza people of Tanzania.[9] There is a remarkable diversity in what these essentially Stone Age people eat. Their diet bears little resemblance to anything you can buy at the supermarket. We have modified our crops and animals so extensively during thousands of years of cultivation that our foods don't resemble their wild ancestors. Size and flavor have changed (this is mostly a good thing) and chemical composition has varied (benefits and drawbacks less clear). Even the meat we eat is totally different in chemical composition. For example, today's meat contains far more omega-6 fatty acids and fewer omega-3 fatty acids than wild meat. And when was the last time you ate internal organs like the kidneys or pancreas, let alone the gut contents, of a freshly killed animal? Moreover, true paleo diets are highly seasonal. For example, at some times of year honey is a major component of the Hadza diet, along with the live bee larvae (which Rob had the opportunity to taste while in Tanzania working with the Hadza in 2014). That said, diets rich in a variety of fruits and vegetables, and in animals that eat their natural diet, have a lot of advantages where they're feasible. But let's not fool ourselves into thinking that we can eat something resembling what hunter-gatherers consume.

But a paleo diet, or the approximation of one you can assemble from your local grocery, does not pose any health problems from a microbiome point of view. To the contrary, like vegetarian and vegan fare, it provides plenty of fiber from fresh vegetables, plus animal protein in meat, fish, and eggs—but forget about the cheese. An exception is farmer's cheese, which resembles the stomach contents of young animals who are still feeding on their mothers' milk. Hunter-gatherers regard this as a delicacy. Olive oil, fruits, and nuts are also fine. Not that our kids don't eat these things. Of course they do. But they also eat other less healthy food, like gummy bears.

How can I make my kid eat foods that are good from a microbiome perspective? Can I trick my picky eater into actually liking those foods?

This is one of the most common questions we get and unfortunately one of the hardest to answer. Fiber exerts the biggest impact on an adult's microbiome, particularly nondigestible carbohydrates—so basically you should eat lots of vegetables and leafy greens. This also holds true for children after they are weaned. But how can you actually get your child to eat a healthy diet? What if your fussy, stubborn toddler only accepts bland foods? Nothing green. Nothing runny. Nothing chewy. Nothing with bits in it like a raisin in a cookie, or one food touching another food on the plate. Yuck.

Jack has friends and colleagues who swear by particular methods, such as introducing fibrous foods early, so that their kid's taste buds get used to them. Both his boys love broccoli and green beans and one of them loves peas. They can sometimes be cajoled into eating lettuce. However, mostly everything else is a fight. He travels a lot and likes to bring along the children. When they are in a foreign country the boys have to eat whatever is available. In China, both have been known to eat simple noodles and rice, and one time they consumed a chicken that was butchered in front of them by a Hani tribal woman, who grabbed the bird off the street, killed it, plucked it, gutted it, and cooked it front of the fascinated boys. They ate it, reluctantly.

But if your kid gravitates toward junk food, you can lay part of the blame on television advertising. In a recent study, twenty-three children between the ages of eight and fourteen were asked to rate sixty food items—half of which were healthy and the other half not—based on how tasty and healthy they looked. Researchers then imaged their brains using functional MRI as they watched junk food ads and nonfood ads. The kids' preference for taste increased after they watched junk food ads and a key decision area of their brains was activated. Junk food images had hijacked their brains. Maybe this is a reason why the American Heart Association recently declared that 91 percent of American children don't have healthy diets.

Jack's son Hayden sometimes seems to survive on mac and cheese. This is a terrible food. It's high-fat and high-sugar. In fact, the starch in the macaroni turns into sugar when it hits the amylase in your child's saliva. So why does he let Hayden eat it? At the end of the day, he's really not living on it. They offer him a balanced diet. He loves raw carrots, will often eat his salad, and downs plenty of fish. One problem is that foods like mac and cheese are commonly found on the kid's menu in restaurants. So it's more of a knee-jerk reaction for him rather than a craving. If they could find more restaurants that offered an array of dishes for kids other than hamburgers, hot dogs, mac and cheese, and grilled-cheese sandwiches, that would be awesome. However, such establishments do not exist in abundance in the United States.

Kids all over the world end up eating a staggering array of foods—herring, kimchi, fried termites, partially digested intestinal contents of a freshly killed gazelle—you name it. Often kids only accept a new food after it's been offered eight to fifteen times. But making your kid eat anything new is a legendary problem and one that neither of us has a good answer for. Maybe one day we will be able to alter a child's microbiome to make them more open to trying new foods—but we are definitely not there yet.

How does sugar affect my child's microbiome?

Sugar has a bad rap. But it tastes so good.

Our bodies are predisposed to crave sugar. This made sense

in the distant past when sugary foods were hard to come by. During our hunter-gatherer beginnings we hunted sweet edibles like honey and fruits because they provided an energy boost. Evolutionarily speaking, those who had greater cravings for such foods may have produced more offspring due to a ready supply of energy. In other words, the theory goes that sugar lovers produced more children and hence helped select for the craving trait within our species. We live with that legacy. The love of sugar is intrinsic to the human psyche, though never more so than in childhood. Jack is persistently amazed by the ability of his boys to consume unfathomable quantities of candy in a single sitting.

But a high-fat, high-sugar diet is not conducive to a healthy gut microbiome. You need fiber, not fried Snickers bars. Or fruit juice, which is also very high in sugar. Simple sugars, like sucrose, can be surprisingly harmful. For example, mice fed a high-sucrose diet were less cognitively flexible. Their ability to switch between thinking about two concepts rapidly—better known as multitasking—is impaired. Bacteria known as *Clostridia* were linked to this observation, and they were significantly more abundant after a diet high in sugar and fat. Importantly, these organisms are known to flourish when the gut is inflamed.

It's possible that a sugary diet could decrease your child's thinking abilities, although, apart from the mouse study discussed above, there is only correlative evidence that kids who eat a lot of sugar have lower attention spans.

Newborns are primed to handle sucrose, which makes sense given that breast milk contains many simple and complex sugars. An infant's early stool often contains bacteria enriched for genes associated with carbohydrate and sucrose metabolism.

People and domestic animals who are obese often have a greater abundance of bacteria that can break down simple sugars.

This is likely because their gut microbes are exposed to much more of it in their diets. Bacteria that use this ample energy resource are likely just responding to its presence in the gut. However, we have evidence that these bacteria may also induce changes in weight gain by themselves.[10] So they may become abundant because of too much sugar in the diet, but once abundant, they can change the way the body stores energy.

Sugar also affects the oral microbiome, promoting the growth of bacteria that reduce the pH on the surface of your child's teeth.[11] This makes their mouth more acidic and leads to the eating away of tooth enamel.

So, should your children consume sugar? Sure, but in moderation. Too much sugar can lead to obesity, inflammation, and rotten teeth.

Can I control my child's weight by changing his microbiome?

Probably, but it's still difficult to figure out exactly how to do it.

It is now quite evident that your child's microbiome can influence weight gain, in part by changing the degree to which his body accesses energy from the foods he eats. But the microbiome also changes circadian rhythms throughout the body, especially the liver, which can lead to shifts in how the body stores energy. A diet heavy in fats and sugars promotes an abundance of gut microbes that are less diverse and no longer have a normal day-to-night rhythm. These bacterial species cause low-grade inflammation and may possibly release chemicals into your child's blood that disrupt how the circadian clock genes work in their liver. This means that the liver perceives time in a completely different way than the brain perceives time. This decoupling causes the body's normal balance, or homeostasis, to be thrown into disarray, and one of the results is increased fat storage.

A diet high in fat and sugar can change children's microbiomes in ways that make it more likely that they will crave such foods, as well as craving more food overall. We don't really understand the specific mechanism behind this yet, but interactions between the immune system, the microbiome, and the brain and the balance of neurotransmitters produced by bacteria in the gut seem to disrupt normal hunger levels, causing a reduction in satiety and an increase in cravings. Since these foods are high in calories, these children are likely to gain more weight than if they don't have those microbial changes. They may even become more lethargic and depressed. Therefore, the number one way to protect kids against obesity is to feed them a healthy diet (and this healthy diet may exert some of its effects through the healthy microbiome it promotes).

But what if your kid is already obese? Or what if he fails to gain weight or becomes anorexic? If that's the case, then, yes, it may be possible to directly alter your child's microbiome either through a fecal transplant, probiotic therapy, or strict changes in diet and lifestyle.

In an intriguing case report, a fecal microbiome transfer caused one normal-weight woman to put on pounds after receiving bacteria from her overweight mother. Although this cannot be relied on as good enough evidence (because it represents a single case in which there were many confounding variables), it suggests that people suffering from chronic weight loss and anorexia might benefit from fecal microbiome transfers. But we still need to perform those experiments. (For more on this, see the work of Dr. Max Nieuwdorp and Dr. Willem de Vos in the Netherlands.) We emphasize that both the FDA and the American Gastroenterological Association have very strict rules for fecal transplantation, and that as of this writing it is only approved for therapy of *C. diff* except in the context of very carefully regulated clinical trials.

Probiotic therapy to reverse weight gain has gained some traction recently, at least in animal models. Mice fed a high-fat diet lost weight after getting a mixture of three probiotics. Their insulin function also improved. We don't yet know if this regime will work for overweight children or adults, but research is underway.

The least invasive way to control weight is, of course, dietary. However, when chubby animals lose weight following a diet, their microbiome still retains a signature of their old body mass, so that when they come off their diet and start eating high-fat, high-sugar food, they are more likely to put on more weight than they had before they started the diet. In fact, for a diet to work, it is necessary to stick with it for nine months, after this time the microbiome signature of obesity starts to decay, and animals are less likely to regain their weight.[12] We know that two mice with the same genes but colonized with different microbes have very different responses to the same food, and the same may be true in humans.

The lesson here is that it takes time for the microbes that underlie weight gain to starve to death in the face of a healthier diet. When they drop below a certain level of abundance, which is not yet well understood and may vary from person to person, they are less likely to cause problems and will be less likely to cause an increase in obesity even if your child eats fatty foods or drink sugary drinks once in a while.

Recently one of our colleagues studied weight gain and loss in children with a rare genetic disorder called Prader-Willi syndrome.[13] Children with this disorder cannot stop eating, to the point where they will hurt people for food. Until now it has been considered purely genetic, but this study provided evidence that microbes are involved. Seventeen children with Prader-Willi syndrome were kept in the hospital and allowed to eat only a diet rich in nondigestible carbohydrates—essentially a high-fiber diet. This caused them to lose weight and changed their microbiomes dramatically. For example, they produced more acetate, a molecule used by other bacteria to make compounds that reduce inflammation by calming the immune system. Interestingly, there is evidence from this study that the children also exhibited an increased ability to control their appetite, although further study is needed to confirm this finding.

The best way to help kids lose weight that we can suggest, at least for now, is to change their diet and control how much they eat. Unlike the Prader-Willi children, most kids won't need to be hospitalized to achieve this, but you'll need to be a strict enforcer.

Do GMOs, pesticide and herbicide residues, artificial sweeteners, or endocrine disruptors like BPA affect my child's microbiome?

To the best of our knowledge, there's no evidence that GMOs (genetically modified organisms that have been designed or manipulated to produce certain characteristics) can affect your child's microbiome in any way. But unlike GMOs, pesticides and herbicides are chemicals that can be harmful. At high enough concentrations they may influence your gut microbiology. In addition, some crops have been genetically programmed to be resistant to certain herbicides, so they are often treated with slightly higher concentration of these compounds.

A recent study out of Stanford found that 38 percent of conventionally grown food contained detectable pesticide residues compared with 7 percent for organic produce.[14] Other studies show that children who eat organic produce have fewer pesticide residues in their urine.[15] However, currently there are no credible studies that have explored the impact of pesticides on the human microbiome. We know of work focused on the impact of arsenic (used as an organic pesticide), but the results have not been peer-reviewed and published.

On the other hand, glyphosate, the active ingredient in the common herbicide Roundup, has been correlated with changes in the animal microbiome.[16] It is a complex molecule that has a bond between carbon and phosphorus, which can only be degraded by enzymes in certain bacteria found in many different environments, from the ocean to the human gut. When these bacteria encounter glyphosate, they break the carbon-phosphorus bond and release a carbon molecule and a phosphate molecule that they then feed on. As the microbes become more abundant, an overgrowth results that could induce immune system changes in the gut, leading to inflammation and possibly even celiac disease. So far much of this is supposition and still needs to be proven in an animal model.

Artificial sweeteners are interesting. Jack used to consume eight to ten cans of diet soda a day. He switched to regular soda only after research suggested that diet soda may be bad for your microbiome and hormone levels.[17] For example, when mice ate fatty foods along with artificial sweeteners, gut bacteria involved in weight gain and glucose intolerance flourished. Interestingly, these problems happened with several different kinds of artificial sweeteners that are chemically very different from one another, suggesting that it might be the sweetness itself that is the problem.

This research raises the possibility that regular consumption of artificial sweeteners may induce a shift in levels of the hormones that control insulin production. The same study demonstrated similar shifts in the human gut microbiome, which could lead to diabetes. So it's probably not a good idea to eat a lot of fatty food and then hope that your diet soda is a saving grace. If you want to drink soda, stick to the sugary stuff. But remember, don't drink too much of it. That's not good for your body either. Of course, the best plan is to eliminate soda entirely.

Finally, many parents worry about a chemical called bisphenol A (BPA), which is found in hard plastics such as baby bottles and the inner lining of most canned goods. It is widely used by the food packaging industry, dentists, opticians, and manufacturers of sports equipment, toys and household electronics. It is ubiquitous in the environment and in human tissue. It is also an endocrine disruptor—a class of molecules that interfere with the production, secretion, transport, action, function, and elimination of natural hormones.[18] BPA mimics estrogen and even causes sex reversal in some species of fish and frogs. Kids are exposed to a lot of it.

Can microbes help? We think so. When rats were fed two bacterial strains commonly found in yogurt (*Bifidobacterium breve* and *Lactobacillus casei*), they had lower levels of BPA in their urine and blood and greater amounts in feces.[19] It looks as if these bacteria are consuming BPA, storing it, and then passing it out of the body in stool.

Evidence is building that bacteria in some common probiotics such as kimchi and kombucha can also reduce the burden of BPA, removing it from your child's body. So there may be some hope in treating BPA toxicity in kids by using bacteria that preferentially take it up and then remove it in the feces. This could be considered analogous to bioremediation, where plants that grow quickly and take up nasty chemicals like arsenic are harvested, burned, and the chemicals destroyed safely. The great thing about bioremediation in the gut is that removal of bad compounds happens naturally. All you have to do is flush them down the toilet.

9

Child Gut

What does my baby's gut look like?

Amazingly, in terms of gut microbes, your infant is like a completely different species from you and other adults. While most of the bacteria in their gut will stay with them throughout their lifetime, the proportions of each species will shift dramatically.[1] Remember that the human gut is an ecosystem, like a rain forest or a prairie. As children grow and as they change the types of food they eat, where they live, and who they live with, their ecosystem changes. As the ecosystem changes, the types of species that proliferate will change.

As we have pointed out, the mode of birth substantially influences the types of bacteria your baby first acquires. Babies born vaginally have microbes that stem from the mother's vagina. Babies born by C-section are more likely to be dominated by species associated with the skin and mouth.[2]

Babies' gut microbiomes soon start to change, depending on the type of food they eat.[3] The bacteria that dominate most infants at four months old use lactate as an energy source, and they require an absence of oxygen. This suggests that their gut is becoming anaerobic and that the bacteria are using the most dominant food substrate, for example, milk.

By twelve months, with the shift to a more adult-like diet, toddlers are generally colonized and dominated by bacteria that are good at consuming fiber. These bacteria produce chemicals used by the child's immune system to regulate inflammation.

We think that the first twelve months of life may be extremely important for helping children's immune systems respond appropriately to all the allergens and antigens that the world is going to throw at them. So having bacteria that produce chemicals to help their body regulate the immune response to these stimulants is incredibly important. Interestingly, infants born by C-section appear to have a significantly different microbiome than vaginally born infants even up to twelve months, where they are dominated by two species which are both fast-growing taxa that like eating sugars.

Between the age of one and three children experience a critical period when their gut microbiomes stabilize.[4] (Their brains undergo a similar critical period of development.) By age three and for most of their adult life, the bacteria in their gut continue reproducing all the time. But here's a surprise. After age three, and despite countless individual differences (at the species level), the overall composition of their microbiome probably doesn't change that much over time. It remains remarkably stable. Jeffrey I. Gordon, at the Washington University School of Medicine, tracked thirty-seven adults over five years.[5] After the first year, 70 percent of their gut bacteria stayed the same; 60 percent were stable over five years.

How is such stability possible? Turnover always happens. But as soon as one bacterium leaves, another is ready to divide and take its place. The initial variability, which is mostly associated with the rapidly changing gut ecosystem in infancy, settles down as the ecosystem settles down. Given a steady diet, your child's immune system will be well-developed by age one. While your child can still acquire different microbes, the ecosystem holds steady, which means that it's hard for new bacteria to colonize the gut. (This is why probiotics are so often ineffective. They can't get a toehold.) Like a robust garden, it is hard for new plants to establish unless we remove some of the other plants or something dramatic happens, like a drought.

Relative to everyone else, your child will have a unique and relatively stable combination of microbes. Unless he experiences a dramatic disturbance (for example, multiple courses of antibiotics or significant dietary changes), his gut microbiome should stay the same—at least with differences that are small compared to the differences between people. But of course, if his gut is disturbed and a pro-inflammatory microbiome takes over, it can become long-lasting in a state of stable dysbiosis. Such a microbiome won't promote health and is not amenable to change. It might require an extra push to escape this rut, such as a course of antibiotics and probiotics or a fecal microbiome transplant to reset the system. It's important to note that most of the evidence for this idea comes from microbiome-based treatments of severe illnesses such as C. *diff*, and that these drastic measures should not be applied without the guidance of a physician.

Importantly, while we know a fair amount about how your kid's gut microbiome develops, we know very little about how the microbiomes in other body sites develop. Very little work has been done. But new research is always being performed to unlock this knowledge. We expect that the skin microbiome will reach stability a lot earlier than the gut, as will the oral and urogenital microbiome. But as your child grows, goes through puberty, and changes his lifestyle, we would expect to see signatures of these events in the microbes that colonize and persist on them.

How do gut microbes shape my child's immune
system?

Our bodies evolved in a world teeming with microbes. They
are in us, on us, all around us—without them, we could not survive. One of the critical jobs they perform is to develop our functional immune system. With it, we fight off disease and further
structure our microbiome by making sure all its elements are in
the right place.

For example, the cells lining your child's gut wall are covered
in a thick mucous layer, much like snot. This goopy layer is home
to some of your child's antibodies, important components of the
immune system that usually identify pathogens by binding to
their surfaces and signaling for white blood cells to come and kill
them. But here's the thing. Most of the antibodies in the mucous
layer bind to the good bacteria in your child's gut—the ones that
keep her healthy.[6] These microbes help regulate your child's inflammatory response by releasing two types of immune cells from
the gut wall that act in an opposing manner. One, called TH17,
promotes inflammation. The other, called Treg, quells it. Obviously you want your child's Tregs (and yours) to stay happy.

The good news is that your child's gut contains bacteria especially designed to feed Treg cells. We've met these kinds of bacteria before. They ferment the fiber or complex carbohydrates in
your diet and release chemicals (those short-chain fatty acids).
When Tregs eat these SFCAs, they release chemicals that stop
TH17 cells from causing inflammation. Pretty neat.

Your child's body relies on these bacterial chemicals to regulate their response to allergens and antigens and to keep their
immune system in balance. Should they overrespond to some
stimulant, they might experience runaway inflammation. We see
this in a condition called sepsis, which occurs in hospitalized

children as well as adults. Their immune system activates inflammation, inviting white blood cells to penetrate tissues and kill off an invading pathogen. But if the immune response is not turned off, inflammation overtakes the body and kills the patient.

Any failure to regulate the inflammatory response in your child's body can have profound consequences for chronic diseases, including food allergies, asthma, and autoimmune conditions ranging from inflammatory bowel disease to diabetes to multiple sclerosis. All of these have now been linked to the gut microbiome.

Gut bacteria also make you and your child less susceptible to infection by forming complex communities that are difficult to invade. Think of it like trying to plant seeds in a mature forest rather than on bare soil: it's hard for the new plants to get a foothold under the canopies of the existing trees. The same principle applies to the microbiome, where the complex interrelationships between the anaerobic microbes that develop over time just don't leave a lot of open ecological niches for new microbes coming in to invade. And this ecological exclusion isn't limited to the bacteria. Recent research shows that even viruses get in on the act by coating the gut lining and then lying in wait, just daring a nasty bacterium to try to infect your body.[7] This is so cool: the virus attacks the attacker and uses it to make more viruses, until the bacterium eventually perishes.

Is the microbiome involved in my child's diarrhea and constipation?

Yes. When your child has diarrhea, stool travels rapidly through her intestines. Depending on the severity of the illness, pretty much everything gets washed out except for certain bacteria that are ecologically adapted to hang on tight.[8] The remaining microbiota have a set of skills designed to help them survive when everything else is flooding through your child's gut. For example, they grow and divide really quickly, so even as many of them get washed out, the same number or more grow and divide. They also manage to feed themselves in the process. Diarrhea reduces the ability of the gut to absorb sugars so the whole gut environment becomes sugary. In turn, the bacteria feed on all that sugar and this powers their rapid growth.

Prevotella, a genus of bacteria found in most healthy guts, feeds on these sugars especially well, so we often see it increasing dramatically during an attack of diarrhea. We also see rapid growth in Proteobacteria such as *E. coli*. The result of these microbial changes is inflammation. Although we don't know the specific mechanism for this, we know that inflammation exacerbates your child's diarrhea. Some pathogens, such as *Salmonella* and *Vibrio cholera* (which causes cholera), promote an immune response that gives rise to so-called reactive oxygen species, molecules that are the bane of many bacteria. Such oxygen-rich molecules burn out other bacteria in the vicinity but leave *Salmonella* and *Vibrio* relatively unscathed.

Diarrhea can also be caused by food intolerance and dehydration, as well as other pathogens such as rotavirus, and parasites like giardia. Each pathogen triggers inflammation by invading your child's gut or releasing toxins into her body. The intestinal tissues then swell, killing off much of the normal gut microbiome and preventing the absorption of water, nutrients, and sugars across the gut wall.

In any case, the main thing is to keep your child hydrated, which means oral rehydration therapy—basically, Gatorade. The sugar in it transports electrolytes across the cells lining your child's gut, and the electrolytes then replace those lost during diarrhea. Obviously, you should use common sense and not allow your child to drink gallons of Gatorade—a quart a day would be ok. Critically, the rehydration therapy won't work without both the salt and the sugar: just giving your baby water (or milk) isn't enough.

Most childhood diarrhea is self-limiting in a few days, but if it persists, is very severe, or your whole family has it, talk to your doctor, because there are many possible underlying causes and some of them are serious.

At the other end of the elimination spectrum, while we know that the gut microbiome differs in patients with constipation versus those without, we still don't fully understand what role the microbiome plays in the problem. People with constipation do not have a reduced abundance of common probiotic strains (such as *Lactobacillus* and *Bifidobacteria*), so probiotic yogurts may not do much good. Until the underlying cause of constipation is better understood, we won't be able to give you advice.

How can I tell if my child has a leaky gut? Can I fix it?

A leaky gut occurs when microbes or microbial products escape your child's gut because a natural barrier has been compromised. This barrier is essentially a layer of epithelial cells that are glued together with so-called tight-junction proteins. Should the glue weaken or the cells become damaged, microbial chemicals or proteins can leak through.

A leaky gut entails runaway inflammation caused by viral proteins or bacterial pathogens that interact with your child's damaged gut wall cells. This, in combination with toxins and other factors, can cause the integrity of the entire gut membrane to break down. All this starts when the mucus that covers the gut wall starts to erode. This layer normally traps a few kinds of beneficial bacteria that cooperate closely with the host cells and keeps the harmful bacteria at bay. It also harbors immune antibodies that control the bacterial population in your child's gut.

When the gut membrane is impaired, bacteria or the chemicals they make can cross more easily into the bloodstream. As noted in the section on oral health and pregnancy, bacteria may get into the bloodstream quite often and are usually dispatched by the immune system. But if your child has hundreds of thousands of bacterial cells crossing over, there will be a huge inflammatory response in the gut wall, runaway inflammation, and possibly sepsis. The microbial chemicals that get into the blood can be innocuous or dangerous. For example, bacterial toxins can make your child very sick. Neurotoxins such as kynurenine can throw the central nervous system out of balance. These conditions are still being investigated.

Although gut barrier dysfunction has been shown in mice under a wide range of conditions and in humans under specific conditions such as liver failure, "leaky gut" is often regarded as a metaphor rather than a direct description of a physical condition. The term became familiar to many parents when the now-debunked measles vaccine and autism controversy exploded in the late 1990s. But there is no evidence that the measles vaccine causes so-called leaky gut.

However, if your physician suspects your child has a gut barrier problem, leaky gut can be diagnosed by several methods. One involves testing the blood for a molecule called LPS, or lipopolysaccharide, which is produced by some kinds of bacteria. When detected, it can indicate that a pathogenic bacterium has gotten into the blood and could cause an infection; most gut bacteria don't make LPS, but the ones that do tend to be more dangerous. The gold standard for finding LPS is to examine cells taken from a slice of the gut. Of course, you'd rather scientists do that to mice instead of your baby.

Another way to test for a leaky gut is to have your child swallow indigestible molecules as markers and see whether and how quickly they end up in the urine. Popular choices are large molecules like polyethylene glycol (PEG) and small sugars such as lactulose and mannitol. One issue with these tests is that the gut sometimes only leaks small molecules, not larger ones. However, it should be possible to determine the degree of leakiness based on the size of the molecule shown to cross the barrier.

Other blood tests look for a protein called zonulin, which correlates with poor barrier function. Another seeks a protein normally used to transport fatty acids within the gut and only detected when it leaks out. Finally, if a marker of intestinal inflammation (calprotectin) and a common serum protein (alpha-1 antitrypsin) are found in the stool, it's likely they leaked into the gut from the bloodstream. These diagnostics are gaining in popularity in adults but haven't been tested much in children.

So if you really want to know if your baby has a leaky gut, looking for the small sugars (testing for lactulose and mannitol) is your best bet. There are downsides: It's expensive. You'll have to starve your kid before feeding her something she won't like. And then you have to collect her urine for hours.

Leaky gut can be fixed by correcting certain vitamin deficiencies, feeding more calories overall, or adding glutamine and micronutrients to your baby's menu. A diet of 25 percent breast milk can help. And if your child has diarrhea caused by bacteria that disrupt the normal gut microbiome, you should try to clear it up.

How do the gut microbiomes of babies and children differ around the world?

Newborns all start off pretty much the same, so the main differences observed in children from around the world involve rates of C-section and antibiotic usage. Both practices tend to reduce microbial diversity in all our kids and affect how their microbiomes develop. However, we are starting to see that one of the most dramatic drivers is poverty.[9] In work from Jack's collaborators at University of Chicago, it has become obvious that in preterm infants who are successfully discharged from the neonatal intensive care unit, the big difference in their microbiomes at age one year, and in their overall health, is whether they are poor.

Poverty can influence the microbiome and human health in many ways: poor diet (especially in the developed world), malnutrition, pollution, and reduced access to health care. We are closely monitoring ways to intervene in the microbial development of infants who are born into poverty to reduce potential health outcomes such as allergies, asthma, and neurological developmental problems such as school readiness.

Where you are born in the world matters.[10] People born in Western urbanized nations have more *Bacteroides* and *Clostridium* in their guts. Those born in underdeveloped regions of Africa and South America show higher levels of *Prevotella*. There are many areas of the world where we still don't have enough data to make a specific statement. In fact, for most countries, not a single person has had his or her microbiome sequenced yet.

We have evidence that human genetics can play a role in shaping the microbiome, but lifestyle, cultural practices, and diet seem to have a much more significant impact.[11] Cultural practices often determine what you eat, and lifestyle affects what you are exposed to. For example, a farmer's children are exposed to more animals early in life; this may be a factor in why they are 50 percent less likely to develop asthma.[12]

These differences in the microbiome in different countries are seen in adults, and we think the same is likely true for infants, except that formula-feeding versus breast-feeding tends to have modest effects. There haven't been a lot of systematic studies of children in different countries using the same methods, so it's often hard to compare results.

We can say that children growing up in more rural environments tend to have more diverse microbiomes and lower rates of allergies and asthma.

Keeping your kids too clean and away from healthy dirt and healthy animals seems to be a problem that triggers a wide range of immune-involved diseases not generally encountered among babies growing up in rural third-world villages. Of course, these children suffer from other problems: limited access to health care and often extremely high rates of maternal and child mortality. So scientists are trying to figure out a happy medium between excellent health care and lifestyle choices, which could influence whether you develop chronic diseases such as autoimmune conditions.

Although identical twins are slightly more similar than nonidentical twins in terms of their adult microbiomes, the effect of their genes is very small.[13] However, a few kinds of bacteria, such as *Christensenella*, match up much better in abundance between identical than nonidentical twin pairs. Intriguingly, when one identical twin is fat and the other is thin, the thin one will have *Christensenella* and the fat one will not. When we take stool from the fat twin and colonize a germ-free mouse, it gets fat. But if we take stool from a fat twin and add *Christensenella* and then colonize a germ-free mouse, the animal does not get fat. Whether any of this applies to our kids remains to be seen in future studies.

10

Depression

I felt depressed before and/or after my baby was born. Were microbes involved?

Pregnancy and childbirth are often hailed as the happiest times in a woman's life. When the "bundle of joy" arrives, it's a period of bliss and falling love with your new baby.

Except when it's not. Between 10 and 20 percent women experience perinatal depression—during the pregnancy and after the baby is born. Prenatal depression can take the form of bouts of crying, sleep problems, fatigue, disturbed appetite, anxiety, and lack of attachment feelings toward your unborn child. Postpartum depression manifests as persistent sadness, fatigue, guilt, mood swings, lack of concentration, and even alienation from the baby. These sensations go far beyond the standard growing pains of parenthood, although this isn't always clear to the sufferers: after Amanda and Rob's daughter was born, Amanda felt suddenly despondent but assumed she was simply adjusting badly to being a new mother. (Fortunately, when their doula stopped by for a follow-up visit, she recognized the telltale signs of postpartum depression and raised the alarm!)

Your chances of developing perinatal depression increase if you have a history of depression or have experienced recent stressful events. But a possible underlying biological explanation has to do with the major hormonal shifts your body undergoes in conceiving, carrying, and giving birth to a baby.

These hormonal shifts change the ways your body produces and uses neurotransmitters. These are the basic currency of your nervous system. They transmit messages between nerve cells, often to speed things up or slow them down. When the delicate equilibrium between speeding up and slowing down the neurons in your brain is disrupted, because of either too much of the transmitters that speed up transmission (for example, serotonin) or too much of the transmitters that slow down transmissions (for example, GABA), you can experience feelings of confusion, depression, and anxiety, and develop other mental health problems.

We used to think that only your brain could produce and use these chemicals, but now we know that gut bacteria produce and consume them as well. That's right. Your gut produces key molecules used in your brain and nervous system. And some recent evidence suggests that when the bacterial community is disturbed, neurotransmitter balance in your body can be profoundly altered.[1]

Gut microbes can affect neurotransmitter balance through a number of metabolic pathways, whereby they produce neuroactive compounds that influence brain development and behavior. These include something called 5-HTP, or 5-hydroxytryptophan, which is an intermediate molecule between the amino acid tryptophan and the neurotransmitter serotonin. It is produced by *Candida*, *Streptococcus*, *Escherichia* and *Enterococcus*. Other bacteria—*Bacillus* and *Serratia*—produce the neurotransmitter dopamine. *Escherichia*, *Bacillus*, *Saccharomyces* make noradrenaline, while *Lactobacillus* can produce acetylcholine. GABA (the neurotransmitter than slows things down) can be produced by both *Lactobacillus* and *Bifidobacterium*.

GABA is also made in the brain, where it acts through GABA receptors that play a role in many kinds of drugs—anxiolytics, hypnotics, general anesthetics, anticonvulsants, and sedatives—and disorders such as epilepsy, multiple sclerosis, depression, and anxiety.

The brain produces serotonin as well, but when a stressful event occurs or hormones go haywire, brain serotonin production can start to plummet for reasons no one fully understands. However, the serotonin produced in the gut can compensate for this loss. Gut serotonin can cross into the brain, where it affects mood, appetite, and feelings of well-being. But 90 percent of this important compound stays in the gut, where it regulates intestinal movements.[2]

Likewise, bacterial GABA has significant impacts on neurotransmitter function through GABA receptors in smooth muscle, epithelium, and endocrine glands, influencing intestinal motility, gastric emptying, acid secretion, sphincter activity, and the sensation of discomfort. But bacterial GABA does not cross the blood-brain barrier and get into the brain, so there's an obvious question as to how it could influence mood.

Clues lie in a superhighway—the vagus nerve—that connects your gut and other vital organs to your brain. Information flows in both directions. Here's how it may work. Some gut bacteria, such as *Lactobacillus brevis* and *Bifidobacterium dentium*, consume the amino acid glutamate to make GABA. Others, such as *Flavonifractor*, eat GABA for their growth. When these bacteria change their activity, the amount of GABA available to your gut's nervous system (sometimes called your second brain) changes. Importantly, the vagus nerve links your gut's nervous system to your brain. If the amount of GABA available goes down, then your gut's nervous system and the vagus nerve can lack the inhibition that keeps the nerve impulses in check. This is felt in your brain through the vagal superhighway.

Also, there are other ways that nerve impulses can get from your gut to your brain. Nerve endings that sense feelings in your stomach and GI tract send signals via your spine up to your brain's insular cortex—a region that monitors and interprets the feeling state of your body. In this way, you can sense the discomforts we mentioned earlier, as well as stomach cramps and pain. As with all nerves in the body, this pathway also uses GABA, so if the amount of GABA is out of balance, your ability to detect these sensations will be affected.

When bacterial GABA interacts with GABA receptors in the vagus nerve or the sensing nerves, pathways that regulate feelings from the body are affected. This in turn seems to alter the balance of GABA being produced and used in the brain, which therefore affects mood. Hence the brain "listens" to the gut. If the gut is upset, then the brain will be too.

And here's where your microbiome comes in. It's plausible that changes in your hormone levels during pregnancy could shift activity of your gut microbes. If you already have a disturbed microbiome and have the potential to be disrupted by hormone changes, then the bacteria that mediate these neurotransmitters will change their activity and you quickly get an imbalance in your body's neurotransmitter concentrations (for example, GABA and serotonin).

What can you do? Can you manipulate your gut microbes to alter neurotransmitter production? It would be a novel therapy for perinatal depression. Unfortunately, the science is just not there yet. We still have a lot to prove. The good news is that the work is proceeding, and if we are right, then it may be possible to just alter your diet or consume some specific bacteria that could rebalance your microbial neurotransmitter activity to actively rebalance your neurological pathways.

I'm worried about getting perinatal or postnatal depression. What can I do?

While you may be able to improve your physical health with diet or probiotics, there's no good evidence that these two strategies can improve your mental well-being.

We know that antidepressants are not the only answer, or at least we're working toward a day when they won't be. Many women worry about taking antidepressants because of the stigma attached to these drugs and the potential harmful side effects, both for mother and baby. Therefore, diet (including omega-3 fatty acid supplementation) and probiotics, which are relatively noninvasive and don't appear to have any side effects (other than over- or undereating), look like favorable alternatives.

A small clinical trial found that probiotics reduced the symptoms of depression and lowered levels of a stress hormone called cortisol.[3] Volunteers participated in a double-blind, placebo-controlled, randomized trial, where a formulation of *Lactobacillus helveticus* R0052 and *Bifidobacterium longum* R0175 (two common probiotics strains you can buy without a prescription) was administered daily for thirty days. Twenty-six people took the probiotic formulation and twenty-nine got the placebo.

After the month was over, doctors assessed each patient's cortisol levels and gave them psychological tests to determine their levels of anxiety and depression. Those taking the probiotics had a significant reduction in psychological distress, including less depression, anxiety, anger, and hostility, and interestingly also showed improved problem solving. However, there was a lot of individual variability, so even though the probiotics in this study worked on average, it doesn't mean they will work for you. It should be noted that the European panel on the substantiation of health claims found major problems with the study, which means the jury is still out on this particular formulation.

Researchers are looking at other species, including some known to alter neurotransmitter levels in human blood. If we know which microbes help alleviate depression, we could make a real difference in many lives.

If I'm depressed, can my baby's microbiome be affected?

Possibly, although right now we just don't know. There are a number of avenues by which this could occur. For example, you pass microbes to your baby through a vaginal birth, skin contact, and kisses. Some of these organisms might cause an imbalance in the production of neurotransmitters in your child's gut, either by suppressing the growth of bugs that produce the neurotransmitters or by actively eating the neurotransmitters and thereby preventing your child's body from accessing them.

The only other obvious way this could happen is if changes in your breast milk chemistry (because of bad diet or bad health) altered the colonization of your baby's gut and resulted in the same problem, specifically an imbalance in the production and consumption of neurotransmitters.

However, there is a surprising gap in research on microbiome and breast milk chemistry and the development of infant mental health. Similarly, there is a significant lack of research into postnatal or postpartum depression—something that Jack's lab is actively trying to address.

Whether a disruption in your microbiome related to postpartum depression could influence your baby's microbiome is just not known.

Depression runs in my family. Can I ward off depression in my child by manipulating his microbiome?

Maybe someday, but you would have to start very early. We have both witnessed depressions in our families. While neither of us suffer from any form of clinical depression, it is most certainly something we have thought about extensively. To date, none of our children have exhibited any symptoms of depression, but the research we and others are doing could help prevent its onset in the future.

We know that the microbiome is linked to depression-like behavior in animals because of some exciting studies performed over the last ten years.[4] These have shown that germ-free mice (which have had all their microbes taken away before birth) have very different risk-taking behavior compared to mice with an intact microbiome. Mice without a microbiome are less anxious and more willing to take risks. Normal mice prefer to hide, which as you might expect is a good thing for a mouse to do in the wild. The mouse that hides stays alive. The mouse that doesn't hide gets eaten. For years we assumed that this risk-avoidance behavior was ingrained in the animals' genome, but the mice in these studies all had the same genome. The only thing that differed was that some of the mice had a microbiome and the others didn't. The mice without a microbiome became "braver" than those with a microbiome. To test this hypothesis further, the researchers added the microbiome from the normal, anxious mice into the guts of the germ-free, brave mice, and lo and behold, the brave mice became anxious and stopped taking risks.

But here's the thing. For mice to start behaving "normally," the bacteria needed to be added back in while the mice were infants. Transplanting the microbiome into adult germ-free mice didn't reverse the behavior. The mice stayed brave and risk-taking.

First, we know what you're thinking. So bacteria cause depression and anxiety? Then surely we need to scrub them out. But that's not only a very bad idea; it's technically impossible in humans. Also, aberrant behavior for a mouse is to be brave and risky, but humans might display different aberrant behaviors. So if we made a germ-free human, it's possible that he or she would be anxious or maybe even depressed.

While anxiety and risk-taking behavior may not seem too close to depression, especially chronic major depressive disorder, the similarities in the mechanisms are probably more common than we once thought. Anxiety and depression are both caused by an imbalance in chemicals in our nervous system that stimulate and inhibit how frequently nerves communicate with each other. Too much stimulation or too much inhibition breaks the delicate balance in our nervous system and leads to aberrant behavior.

Importantly, these studies also suggest that these behaviors that we once thought were grounded in the genome may actually be coded into our microbiome. This means that depression could be transmitted from parent to offspring, not by the human genes but by the bacterial genes in the microbiome.

The question remains: why doesn't this kind of microbiome manipulation work in adult animals?

If humans are anything like mice (and we have plenty in common), the brain is malleable for a critical period in infancy and childhood, even into adolescence. The plasticity of the brain and nervous system decreases with age. So changing the microbiome in infancy may be the only way to influence the development and structure of the brain. If you have a family history of depression, you may need to add the right kind of microbes into your child's gut during this critical period. We don't know exactly what the right kind of microbes are or what the right time frame is, but it could be as early as during pregnancy or in the earliest weeks of life.

We have started to examine the microbiomes of people who are depressed and those who are not, and yes, they are different.[5] For example, depressed people have a reduction in bacteria that produce neurotransmitters, especially GABA and the precursor of serotonin. Using this strategy, we might develop probiotics with these bacteria to treat depression. But before we try them in humans, we need to test them in animals, and that takes time and patience—a lot of patience.

Before we start giving our infants probiotics, we need to be aware of how they will respond. The problem is that infants' immune systems are very sensitive. Adding the wrong set of microbes could cause a massive inflammatory response, and this could affect how the brain develops as well. It is not simple. Many things can go wrong. Excessive inflammation could even retard brain development and cause any number of mental health problems. An immature brain is more susceptible to altered development. It means we need to be careful in determining which bacteria to select as probiotics. Remember, a probiotic should be health-promoting, so a bacterium that causes developmental problems would not be a probiotic.

Is my child's microbiome linked to his learning difficulty?

To be honest, we don't know. When scientists conduct studies looking for links between something like learning disorders or school readiness and early-life microbial development, we usually pick worst-case scenarios. This allows us to see relationships through the lens of extreme responses.

For example, each year 1 percent of babies in the United States are born prematurely and classified as extremely low birth weight infants, weighing less than 2.2 pounds. We have gotten very good at helping these kids, so now 78 percent of them survive. Yet there are complications. Such infants have very high rates of mental disability and up to 40 percent of them score low on cognitive tests, meaning they have problems acquiring knowledge and understanding their world through thought and experience.

While it is easy to say that their brains were born too early, and that this is an unavoidable problem with preterm birth, the facts don't support this conclusion. Neither gestational age nor birth weight predicts long-term neurological developmental problems in children. We know that some complications—such as lung damage caused by excessive ventilation with high oxygen, obvious brain injury, seizures, diabetes, and necrotizing enterocolitis where the bowel starts to die—are associated with poor neurological development. However, most of these are also associated with inflammation, and some experts have hypothesized that the microbiome could play a role in controlling these conditions.

Remember that preterm infants are given extensive rounds of antibiotics, so their microbiome is very disturbed. Practices such as breast-feeding, which restore that balance, can have a positive outcome on neurodevelopment. Therefore, perhaps, any element that supports a healthy microbiome, even in preterm infants, could help prevent the onset of learning difficulties later in life.

Socioeconomic status also plays a role in neurodevelopment and learning. Preemies who leave the neonatal intensive care unit with the same degree of cognitive development can have very different outcomes. Those going home to disadvantaged households are less ready for school at age five compared to babies raised in wealthier homes. Although at age two both groups of kids have normal cognitive development, by elementary school only 8 percent of the better-off kids required special education, compared to 29 percent of those less well-off.

You might dismiss these disparities as a function of access to good preschools and elementary school education, but large-scale studies show those correlations just don't hold water. Jack's lab is taking a closer look at how an infant's microbiome develops between six and eighteen months of age. Children born into a lower socioeconomic homes generally have diets richer in saturated fats and sugar, and have less access to animals and natural environments (especially in urban settings). It's possible that these issues may interfere with the infant's neurological development by affecting the balance of gut bacteria that produce neurotransmitters and cause excess inflammation, which can also retard brain development.

Interestingly, malnutrition can also cause neurodevelopmental problems. In animal studies, malnutrition-induced changes in the microbiome have been shown to reduce cognition—independent of the malnutrition itself.

The research is still in progress, so we cannot honestly say whether these hypotheses will hold out. But bear in mind that if these concerns are true, then it may be possible to develop probiotics or forms of microbial medicine to help children have a better neurological developmental trajectory. Essentially, this means we might build better brains.

11

Vaccines

Are vaccines safe for infants?

From a public health perspective, vaccines have likely saved more lives than any other medical advance. (The other contenders are improved sanitation, antibiotics, and the "green revolution" that dramatically reduced famine around the world.) In a world without vaccines, the polio virus can kill children or paralyze them for life. Measles can lead to brain swelling, lung infection, and death. Even chicken pox, generally thought of as benign, can produce bleeding disorders, infected blisters, and swollen brains and lungs.

When Rob was a kid, his parents explained to him that it was actually good that he was getting chicken pox over Christmas and not later as an adult, when the risk of hospitalization and death from chicken pox is much higher. But it was extremely itchy and uncomfortable—so much so that one of his younger brothers, who got it at the same time, still has a scar on his face from scratching so hard. Fortunately, this unpleasant milestone of childhood can now be retired: like many American children,

Rob's daughter was fully vaccinated against chicken pox before she was two years old.

Compared to the havoc caused by viral infections, vaccines are incredibly safe. Yes, rare adverse reactions can occur. These are mostly limited to swelling, redness, itching, sometimes headaches, fatigue, and nausea; but life-threatening allergic responses to vaccines are extremely rare. Compared to the diseases we're talking about, the risks posed by vaccines are far lower than the risks of contracting an infection.

We now know that probiotics can influence the effectiveness of a vaccine. But we don't yet know if your child's microbiome by itself might influence a vaccine's effectiveness. Since a healthy microbiome can make your child's immune system more alert, it could improve the outcomes of a vaccine.

We understand why people may be worried about giving their child a vaccine. There is a huge amount of negative information circulating on the Internet and on playgrounds across the country. When someone you trust tells you that vaccines can hurt your child, you naturally ask yourself if you should believe them.

While you may not be ready to trust us, we hope you will consider the expertise and experience of the nation's board-certified pediatricians. "High immunization rates are critical for keeping disease outbreaks at bay," writes Dr. Benard P. Dreyer, president of the American Academy of Pediatrics (AAP), in a recent report published in the journal *Pediatrics*. "No child should have to suffer through a disease that could have been prevented by a vaccine."[1] Yet more and more of them are: Whooping cough is resurgent in the United States, infecting tens of thousands of babies—the most reported number of cases since 1955.

The AAP report explains that nearly all the bad things you have heard have no validity for the vaccines your child will get today. There used to be a chemical present in the carrier fluid in vaccines prior to 1998 that was associated with some health problems, but this has been removed from all vaccines and no longer poses a threat (if indeed the limited studies supported it as actually dangerous). We can state categorically that we have reviewed the evidence, and apart from extremely rare allergic reactions, there are no obvious risks associated with vaccines but tremendous benefit proven in thousands of studies and in countries around the world.

Kids get sick frequently, and there are many anecdotes about children becoming ill after getting a combined vaccine shot. But this does not mean the vaccine caused the illness. Our kids had the full MMR vaccination, and both of Jack's kids had mild lethargy and a short period of elevated temperature post-vaccination. Also, Jack's oldest son had a number of yeast infections around the time he was supposed to get the MMR, so his parents waited until they had cleared up before administering the vaccine. These are things your doctor will tell you if you talk to them. Honestly, you should voice your concerns. Among all the clinical scientists and medical practitioners we work with, we have never come across any instance of a pharmaceutical company influencing them to prescribe a vaccine.

One important exception to the efficacy of vaccines concerns infants who are too young to respond because they don't have fully formed immune systems: in this case, the vaccines will not form antibodies to the pathogen you want to ward off. The CDC vaccination schedule is organized so that vaccines are administered when they will be effective. In general, the earlier your child is vaccinated the better, because that reduces the amount of time he is unprotected. But there is also an ideal age when your child's immune system will work best for each vaccine.

Parents often ask us about the scheduling of all those shots.

Is it better to give them in one go or to space them out over time? There's no simple answer, though many vaccines need to be given in repeated doses over time to make the immune response as strong as possible. But why are twenty-five shots recommended in the first fifteen months of life? Why not spread them out over two or three years? The answer is that you would not want your child to go unprotected that long. A first exposure to the measles or polio virus at age three or four could be disastrous. Plus there is no scientific evidence to support a shorter schedule. And there's no way to test your child for natural immunity to this or that disease because these assays don't work well for young children.

However, it may one day be possible to identify the best time to vaccinate your child based on how his individual microbiome matures. As we discussed in the child gut section, your child's microbiome undergoes a developmental trajectory. Although there is significant variability in the details of this trajectory, most children follow a similar path. Since we know that the microbiome influences the effectiveness of a vaccine, it may one day be possible to sequence your child's microbiome to determine the optimal timing for getting the shots. Right now, we don't know what that ideal might look like, but it could be based on individual microbes or collections of specific microbes that support the immune system. Unfortunately, we can't yet test infants and children quickly and on a large scale for variations in their immune systems based on variations in their gut microbes. But it's a goal we have in mind.

. . . .

Our basic message in this book has an intrinsic complication that we'd like to further explore. We've advised you to embrace microbial diversity while protecting your child from exposure to pathogens. Let's take a closer look at this dichotomy.

First, pathogens. Their constant presence throughout human evolutionary history shaped our immune system to expect to encounter them at all times without warning. You never knew when you'd come into contact with a nasty bug and its virulent antigens. (An antigen is any substance that causes an immune system to produce antibodies against it.) So we evolved hypervigilant immune systems prepared to do battle with any and all pathogens. For example, tuberculosis has been around for thousands of years, and people who survived the infection probably developed robust immune responses that were passed down through generations.

When we remove pathogens from our world with vaccines, better sanitation, and the like, we encounter unintended consequences. Our immune systems begin to overreact to things that are not so dangerous—such as pollen or other allergens. This raises a question: should we get rid of vaccines to prevent allergic diseases? If we did away with vaccines, what would happen?

A nonscientific experiment is underway all across the United States that may possibly answer those questions. Many parents have come to believe that we coevolved with childhood diseases over thousands or millions of years and that this means we can accommodate them. In other words, diseases like measles, mumps, and whooping cough are not all that bad. One reason these parents don't fear childhood diseases like measles and polio is that they've never encountered them. These diseases are brutal and lethal. Vaccines have eliminated the scourges that were rampant from the seventeenth through the twentieth centuries, claiming millions of lives. We should be profoundly grateful that we have vaccines against them.

Yet parents who don't understand this history have coalesced into a vocal community that is ardently opposed to vaccines. They cite hazardous ingredients in the formulations and argue that children get too many shots too soon. Not surprisingly, measles, mumps, and whooping cough have made a huge comeback in schools across the United States. Whether these kids will be protected from allergies may never be known because this sort of "experiment" is highly disorganized and, in our opinion, unethical.

One thing more to consider is that vaccines expose your child's immune system to only the specific pathogens you want to protect them from. Modern vaccines are specific: they don't affect the rest of your child's microbes. So unless there's some reason we don't know about as to why a child must experience a major infection in order to activate some later health benefit, you should definitely vaccinate your children. Vaccinating your child has additional benefits: infectious diseases require a certain fraction of the population to be susceptible to new infections so that they can spread, so when most people are vaccinated this "herd immunity" prevents even the few individuals who can't be vaccinated, such as those with severe immune deficiencies or who the vaccine doesn't work on, from getting sick. The alternative could be catastrophic not just for your kids but for everyone.

Is there a schedule for taking vaccines that will best protect my child, and should I consider his microbiome when choosing this?

Babies and children should get their vaccines on the schedule provided by the American Academy of Pediatrics and the Centers for Disease Control and Prevention. Based on the combined data of hundreds of clinical trials, it's your best guide to making sure your child avoids a number of serious bacterial and viral diseases.

Table 2 lists childhood diseases and their respective vaccines. As you will see, many of the complications of these diseases can

TABLE 2. PREVENTABLE DISEASES AND THEIR RESPECTIVE VACCINES

Disease	Vaccine	Method of Spread	Symptoms	Complications
Chicken pox	Varicella vaccine	Air, direct contact	Rash, tiredness, headache, fever	Infected blisters, bleeding disorders, encephalitis (brain swelling), pneumonia
Diphtheria	DTaP vaccine	Air, direct contact	Sore throat, mild fever, weakness, swollen glands in neck	Swelling of the heart muscle, heart failure, coma, paralysis, death
Haemophilus influenzae type b	Hib vaccine	Air, direct contact	May be no symptoms unless bacteria enter the blood	Meningitis (infection of the covering around the brain and spinal cord), intellectual disability, epiglottitis (life-threatening infection that can block the windpipe and lead to serious breathing problems), pneumonia, death
Hepatitis A	HepA vaccine	Contaminated food or water, direct contact	May be no symptoms; otherwise, fever, stomach pain, loss of appetite, fatigue, vomiting, jaundice (yellowing of skin and eyes), dark urine	Liver failure, arthralgia (joint pain), kidney, pancreatic, and blood disorders
Hepatitis B	HepB vaccine	Contact with blood or body fluids	May be no symptoms; otherwise, fever, headache, weakness, vomiting, jaundice (yellowing of skin and eyes), joint pain	Chronic liver infection, liver failure, liver cancer

(continued)

TABLE 2.

Disease	Vaccine	Method of Spread	Symptoms	Complications
Influenza (Flu)	Flu vaccine	Air, direct contact	Fever, muscle pain, sore throat, cough, extreme fatigue	Pneumonia
Measles	MMR vaccine	Air, direct contact	Rash, fever, cough, runny nose, pinkeye	Encephalitis (brain swelling), pneumonia, death
Mumps	MMR vaccine	Air, direct contact	Swollen salivary glands, fever, headache, tiredness, muscle pain	Meningitis (infection of the covering around the brain and spinal cord), encephalitis (brain swelling), inflammation of testicles or ovaries, deafness
Pertussis (whooping cough)	DTaP vaccine	Air, direct contact	Severe cough, runny nose, apnea (a pause in breathing in infants)	Pneumonia, death
Polio	IPV vaccine	Air, direct contact, through the mouth	May be no symptoms; otherwise, sore throat, fever, nausea, headache	Paralysis, death
Pneumococcus	PCV vaccine	Air, direct contact	May be no symptoms; otherwise, pneumonia (infection in the lungs)	Bacteremia (blood infection), meningitis (infection of the covering around the brain and spinal cord), death
Rotavirus	RV vaccine	Through the mouth	Diarrhea, fever, vomiting	Severe diarrhea, dehydration
Rubella	MMR vaccine	Air, direct contact	Rash, fever, swollen lymph nodes	Very serious in pregnant women: can lead to miscarriage, stillbirth, premature delivery, birth defects
Tetanus	DTaP vaccine	Exposure through cuts in skin	Stiffness in neck and abdominal muscles, difficulty swallowing, muscle spasms, fever	Broken bones, breathing difficulty, death

be very serious, and may even include death. Readers should know that both of us have had our children fully vaccinated using the vaccine schedule recommended by the CDC, which you can find at www.cdc.gov/vaccines/schedules/downloads/child /0-18yrs-schedule.pdf.

Should I give my child probiotics before or after vaccination?

Possibly. Studies show that probiotics can be helpful before and after vaccination. Vaccines are agents that resemble disease-causing microbes, but they are carefully designed to be safe. They are often weakened or killed forms of the microbe, a microbial toxin, or a single protein from the microbe (such as one from its surface that is then easily spotted by your immune system when the microbe attacks you later). When your child is given a vaccine, his immune system is activated to recognize the microbe, disable it, and make a memory so that the bug can be destroyed much faster in any future encounter.

Probiotics have been shown to make vaccines more effective. For example, *L. rhamnosus* GG and *L. acidophilus* CRL431 can improve your child's response to polio vaccine by stimulating his immune system.[2] Similarly, a study performed in Singapore fed seventy-seven infants a probiotic cocktail (*B. longum* and *L. rhamnosus* LPR) and compared the efficacy of a hepatitis B vaccine to a placebo control group of sixty-eight infants who didn't get the probiotic.[3] The infants who got the probiotic showed a significant increase in their immune response to the vaccine, suggesting improved effectiveness. We see a similar response in animal studies for the flu vaccine. The basic idea is that microbes can stimulate the immune system making it more alert to the vaccine. The more alert it is, the faster and better it can produce antibodies to the vaccine's antigen.

However, there are other studies that find probiotics do little or nothing to improve the efficacy of vaccines. This is a challenge with all clinical trials. There are so many things that could influence the result. It can be very hard to understand why an intervention worked well in one group and not in another.

To make matters more confusing, an Australian study with sixty-one women examined what would happen if they consumed probiotics late in their pregnancies.[4] Thirty-one took a probiotic (*Lactobacillus rhamnosus* GG) and thirty took a placebo (maltodextrin) every day from week thirty-six of gestation until delivery. The researchers vaccinated their children at age one against tetanus, *Haemophilus influenzae* type b (Hib), and viral pneumonia. Strikingly, the effectiveness of the vaccine was actually reduced in infants whose mothers ate probiotics during pregnancy. So maybe probiotics might not be a good idea after all. However, this was a small study, and although the effectiveness of the vaccine was reduced, the total immune response in the children to the vaccine antigen was not influenced.

In another study performed in Finland, forty-seven women took a probiotic cocktail during their pregnancies, containing four types of beneficial bacteria (*L. rhamnosus* GG, *L. rhamnosus* LC705, *B. breve* Bbi99, and *Propionibacterium freudenreichii* ssp. shermanii JS.) The women were chosen for the study because their infants were at an increased risk of developing allergies.[5] At least one parent had clinically diagnosed allergic rhinitis, atopic dermatitis, or asthma. Forty mothers from this same group were given a control placebo composed of an inert substance.

After birth, the infants whose mothers ate the probiotic were given the same mix in twenty drops of sugar syrup also containing a prebiotic every day for six months. The forty placebo infants were given just the sugar syrup without the prebiotic or the probiotics.

At six months of age, all infants were vaccinated against diphtheria, tetanus, and Hib. The probiotic seemed to make the influenza vaccine more effective and did not decrease the effectiveness of the other two. The authors argued that microbial biomass in an infant's gut is important for diversifying and expanding the repertoire of antibodies. This makes sense because a diverse microbiome would produce a diverse array of antibodies. However, we still don't understand exactly why the probiotic would improve the vaccination efficiency of only one of the three vaccines.

Nevertheless, a probiotic after any vaccine challenge may be good for your child. Piglets were exposed to rotavirus, which causes acute gastroenteritis, and then treated with *L. rhamnosus* GG and *B. lactis* Bb12.[6] They experienced significantly less diarrhea and gut inflammation compared to animals not given the probiotics. It appears the probiotics helped stabilize their guts and supported their bodies in accepting the vaccine.

One thing for sure, these studies point to the notion that gut microbial composition can influence how vaccines work—but as of yet we have no consensus on which probiotics you should take during pregnancy or give to your child to help improve his responsiveness to the vaccine. However, rest assured that there is a lot of ongoing research in this area.

Should my child get a flu shot?

Yes, assuming he's old enough. One flu vaccine is recommended for anyone over six months old, although others are not given until age three or are even restricted to adults. You'll need to talk to your pediatrician to discuss what's best for your child. That said, young children are not immune to the serious risks and complications that are associated with flu. Flu rates are higher in children, and yet the classic symptoms (fever, sore throat, tiredness, and tissue pain) are often invisible, especially in young infants. Most kids tend to vomit and have diarrhea instead of the weakness and stuffy heads seen in adults. We all know that kids are germ factories (that's what we are constantly told, right?), and in kids, flu is infectious for almost twice as long as it is in adults. Flu complications in children include viral pneumonia, bacterial pneumonia, ear infections, brain-associated disorders including seizures, and even death.

The flu is not the same as the common cold. Different viruses cause them. Influenza A and B affect people differently compared to more common rhinoviruses. The flu can make you wish the world would go away. The common cold mostly makes your nose run.

The bacteria in your gut might be able to improve the effectiveness of the flu vaccine.[7] But so far, all the evidence is from a study done in our favorite animal model, the mouse. As we have pointed out in many entries, the microbiome plays a prominent role in stimulating your immune system. Here, the bacteria stimulate the immune system to more efficiently make antibodies to the flu vaccine. Unfortunately, we can't yet recommend which bacteria you should have in your gut to improve your immune response. In this animal study they used a particular strain of *E. coli* to stimulate the immune system's response to the flu vaccine.

Bottom line: everyone in your household, including you, should get flu shots.

12

Environment

Shouldn't I be afraid of germs?

The notion that germs are dangerous has been ingrained into our social consciousness for a very long time. This is understandable if you remember how we discovered these organisms. First observed in the seventeenth century with primitive microscopes, they did not become controversial until the nineteenth century when these "little animals" that we now call bacteria were linked to disease.

The flamboyant and brilliant French scientist Louis Pasteur demonstrated the connection when he proved the idea of germ theory. He argued that the tiny seeds of microbes that floated in the air and landed in the wounds of soldiers were the foundation of disease. The pus that was emitted by their festering wounds was caused by microbial germs. What followed was 150 years of a nearly universal view that germs were bad. They had to be wiped out to keep humans healthy. This made sense since bacteria were killing millions of people each year in the United States and Europe alone. The desire to find ways to eliminate these invaders, or protect us against them, was paramount. The idea pervaded our consciousness and the consciousness of generations to follow. We became a kill-them-all society, where the only good bacteria were dead bacteria.

Ironically, it was Pasteur who wrote, "An animal's existence would be impossible without microbial life." Our destinies are so intertwined that there can be no separation. To sunder these two life forms would result in the death of the host—namely, us.

It turns out that this view—that we cannot live without our germs—is not entirely correct. In the 1920s, scientists figured out a way to breed mice in special sterile chambers. The mice are born germ-free. This is not a natural phenomenon: no such mice could come into existence in the real world. When taken out of their chambers, they are highly susceptible to airborne bacteria and viruses as well as germs carried by their handlers. They often turn septic and die. But if they stay in their box, they thrive. (We scientists use them for many kinds of experiments involving microbial transfers and other types of manipulation.) But here's the thing. These germ-free animals were the first to demonstrate that survival in the real world depends on acquiring trillions of microbes at the start of life. A new theory was born: the radical idea of "good" bacteria.

The probiotic industry got started around the same time. A few scientists began to argue that certain foods containing living organisms could prolong life. It was a way of combating the bacterial menace. Embrace microorganisms that appear to bolster health and development and you win the battle.

Those two worlds, the antibiotic and probiotic, have now existed side by side for six generations. But today, for the first time, they are being blended. We are realizing that the antibiotic strategy can take us only so far and has many unintended consequences. We still need to kill pathogens, but we also need to embrace the good bacteria to balance the equation.

So yes, this means dirt is good. Mud pies rule.

Can the germs on diapers hurt my baby?

From a microbiome perspective, we have no data, just common sense.

Regarding water use and waste disposal, diapers are a controversial topic—cloth or disposable? If you live in a place with water shortages, the environmental cost of using local water to wash cloth diapers may be higher than water usage at the plant where the disposable diapers are made.

In terms of where your baby's fecal microbes end up, disposables go to the landfill, which is likely well isolated from groundwater sources. As for cloth, your city's water treatment infrastructure is set up to handle high levels of feces from everyone flushing their toilets (so you probably haven't had a cholera epidemic lately).

In terms of your child's health, the tiny traces of microbes on new paper products, including diapers, and left over on your cloth diapers after you wash them with detergents, pale into insignificance compared to the high levels of microbes coming directly from your baby's body. In other words, it's hard to imagine that your diapers have more microbes on them than your baby's actual poop, and if they did you should certainly switch brands immediately.

How can I help my child build up a healthy immune system and microbiome that resists disease? Is it different for resisting infectious versus chronic diseases?

This is an important question and an active area of research. Right now the prevailing understanding is that your child needs the right mixture of protection from disease as well as exposure to a rich microbial environment. This balance is complex, and we have discussed these issues in detail in other sections.

We strongly recommend that your child be vaccinated; this is a way to strengthen her immune system against dangerous pathogens. But what else can you do? How can you reduce the likelihood of your child suffering from seasonal allergies or food allergies? What about asthma and other conditions?

Well, the short answer is, let your kids experience as much microbial diversity as you can find. Get them outside, let them interact with animals, allow them to play in the dirt, rivers, streams, ocean. Don't sterilize everything they are going to touch or put into their mouth. A great example of this is the pacifier that falls on the ground. Parents who sterilize the binky run the risk of increasing the likelihood that their child will develop food sensitivities later in life.[1]

But exactly how does exposure to dirt, dogs, and donkeys build a healthy (strong) immune system early in life?

Infants first come into contact with our wildly diverse microbial world when they pass through the birth canal. While in the womb, they acquire some antibodies from your body via the placenta (called passive immunity), but these are designed to help the babies' bodies recognize and fight off dangerous infections before they can produce their own antibodies. We have preliminary evidence that some of these antibodies might also help your baby to start structuring and retaining her early microbiome. Not all antibodies are designed to label bacteria for immune cell execution: some are there to recognize good bacteria and keep them in the right place in your infant's body.

Your baby soon comes into contact with thousands of other types of bacteria, viruses, fungi, and protists (microscopic organisms with cells that have nuclei, like ours, but that are not animals or plants or fungi—it's complicated.) Your baby's immune system soon starts to learn about these bugs—to recognize them. Some of the microbes become part of her body's self-defense mechanism—the microbiome—helping to break down allergenic proteins and compounds that could cause the immune system to go on full alert. They also produce chemicals that feed the immune system and stop it from overreacting. This partnership is highly dynamic, and we are still working furiously to try and understand its complexity.

Importantly, though, early microbiome exposure and development play a pivotal role in educating children's immune systems, helping them to fight off acute and chronic diseases for the rest of their lives.

Should I take my kids to a farm?

Yes, as early in their life as possible, and as frequently as possible. And while there, let them stroke as many animals as they want and even rub their faces up against the ones that will let them. Let them enjoy all the dirt, mud, grit, and dust they can find. Rolling in hay won't hurt. Feeding critters by hand is fun. The only word of caution is that you might want to stop them from eating any poop they find on the floor. Some animals, especially pigs, reptiles, and amphibians, carry parasites or bacteria that could make your kids sick (and not just in their poop but also on their skin).

Our ancestors chose to domesticate certain animals: dogs for hunting and guarding; cows for milk and meat; pigs, chickens, goats, horses, and cats for filling an array of needs. We are descended from those herders, farmers, and horsemen whose choices of which animals to bring into their fields, corrals, and homes helped shape their immune function—and, as distant relatives, that of you and your children.

When young children interact with domesticated animals, they are exposed to a huge diversity of outdoor bacteria that help tutor their developing immune systems; this is why you should visit farms if at all possible.

Children who grow up on farms have a lower likelihood of developing asthma and allergies.[2] Unlike children glued to their iPads, kids who play a lot outdoors are thoroughly exposed to pollen, plants, soils, and ambient bacteria. They, too, show fewer allergic reactions.

Interestingly, in the late nineteenth century, hay fever was common among the British and American upper classes. But farmers, who came into contact with more animals and plants—not so much. Then in Switzerland in the 1990s, scientists identified the "farm effect." Kids who grew up on farms were between a half and a third less likely to have hay fever and asthma compared to city kids. Abundant microbes found in cowsheds conferred protection on farm kids.[3]

We can relate. As a kid, Jack kept rats, turtles, newts, frogs, snakes, stick insects, a dog, lizards—and gerbils kept in their own outdoor autonomous network of tunnels. Rob had terrariums with frogs, lizards, snakes, turtles, and salamanders, while his family had chickens, cats, rats (yes, on purpose), a dog, and even a deer caught in the wild. Though we didn't know why it was important at the time, we loved being exposed to their exotic bacteria.

The theory that exposing your kid to the natural world is worthwhile is known as the "hygiene hypothesis." The theory, which is often expounded by our colleague Erika von Mutius, suggests that children's environment can be "too clean" to effectively stimulate or challenge their immune system.

When scientists first started to tease apart the hygiene hypothesis, they found tight correlations between the likelihood of a child developing an allergy or asthma and the number of plant and animal species found within one mile of his or her home. Local biodiversity seems to play a role in mediating your child's immune experience. In other words, the fewer allergens around, the more likely kids would develop allergies.

Erika's work, among many others, went on to demonstrate that it is not just the number of animals and plants that your child is exposed to but the number of bacteria that live on them. This sort of microbial complexity helps to provide a credible explanation behind the hygiene phenomenon. Children who grow up with exposure to a diverse array of bacterial species, as is found in different animals, will have their immune experience shaped by these bugs. The greater the diversity of these bacteria, the better.

When we look for groups of people today with the lowest rates of immune dysfunction, we find it among people who still directly interact with domesticated animals. A child growing up with a dog will have a 13 percent reduction in the likelihood of developing asthma, which seems remarkable when you remember that the majority of immunologists associated with asthma therapy regard dogs as "causes" of the disease, or at least active exacerbations, rather than protectors. Similarly, those growing up on a farm will have a 50 percent reduction in the likelihood of developing asthma, for many of the same reasons.

In our own work with Erika and other colleagues, we have come across a number of interesting vignettes that highlight this concern. When we compare the Amish and Hutterites, two religious communities in the United States that reject modern conveniences for a simpler, technology-limited life, we find a fascinating difference. The Amish have very low rates of asthma in their population, while the Hutterites have asthma rates four to five times the U.S. average.[4] The only real difference between these two populations is lifestyle choice. Both descend from the same eastern European ancestral populations that have lived an agrarian lifestyle for many generations. Genetically there are no differences that could explain this dichotomy.

So what went wrong? Well, the Amish live on family farms, where the children grow up extensively interacting with the farm environment. They work when their parents work, they all help out with the pigs, cows, and sheep. Even as infants they are often strapped to one of their parents as mom and dad do the rounds on the farm.

The Hutterite children have a different experience. For cultural reasons, as well as practical concerns, their children today are not allowed on the farm. The Hutterites live on big communal properties, with the dwellings arranged around a central farm. The men and boys over the age of fourteen are picked up each morning and driven out to the farm to work the animals and fields. The Hutterites also employ far more mechanization on their property than the Amish—but that still couldn't explain these differences. The absence of the early-life exposure to animals among the Hutterites is one highly probable trigger for their elevated levels of asthma. While their European ancestors were exposed to all the bacteria and allergens found on farms and developed robust immune systems as a consequence, their American-born descendants have deprived their infants and children of the same experience.

In this study we also confirmed the hygiene phenomenon by exposing mice who were susceptible to asthma to household dust from the two farming environments and determining whether it affected their chance to developing asthma. Remarkably, the dust and microbes from the Amish homes were protective and the dust and microbes from the Hutterite homes were not.

Modern life is very comfortable. Children don't have to work. Chores are often minimal and limited to jobs that protect our kids from exposure to dangerous diseases. This has worked out well for us. Public health measures have played a major role in reducing infant mortality and the spread of diseases within our population. Measures such as clean water and good sanitation are not as targeted as vaccines to specific pathogens (and vaccines protect us even when we are exposed to bad germs rather than preventing exposure), but nevertheless they are effective. But this intervention, this separation of our bodies from the real and imaginary dangers of the world, has also severed us from exposures to benign and less harmful bacteria that our ancestors got used to experiencing.

That's why these trips to a farm, or even—if possible—engaging in local farming projects or gardening, can be so vital. It adds back in a little bit of that experience. With proper vaccination and with attention to basic infectious disease principles about what is likely to contain potentially pathogenic organisms (don't eat pig feces, don't handle raw or rotting meat and then put your hands in your mouth, etc.), your children should be free to explore the world, getting nice and dirty in the process.

Should I get a dog?

Yes, and the earlier the better. You may notice that your baby crawls relentlessly toward most any dog that comes within reach. Part of the reason is that humans have long had an innate fascination with canines. We've bred them into hundreds of breeds, and we happily adopt mutts of all shapes, colors, and sizes.

It's win-win. We give them food, shelter, exercise, affection. They give us gobs of love, companionship, hours of play, and valuable services. (Someone is at the front door! Let me fetch that sheep. You want truffles? I will find them for you.)

But there is also an invisible relationship between you and your dog that you may not have noticed. Every time your pooch trots back into your house, it brings bacteria from the outside, thus increasing the diversity and number of microbes to which your baby is exposed. This may sound alarming but it's actually a good thing.

Your child's developing immune system interacts with those bacteria and is better off for it.[5]

Researchers recently cultured a lactobacillus bacterium from dogs, gave it to mice that suffered from asthma, and then saw a significant reduction in the likelihood of the mice having an asthmatic attack.[6] This observation may explain why children growing up with dogs have a 13 percent reduction in the likelihood of developing asthma and allergies.[7]

Another study we mentioned earlier from Rob's lab recruited sixty families with and without children and dogs.[8] Seventeen of them had kids between six months and eighteen years. Another seventeen had dogs but no children. Eight families had both kids and dogs, while eighteen families had neither. Amazingly, dog ownership significantly increased the number of bacteria shared by the couples who kept them in their homes. It appears that dogs increase the transmission of bacteria in the household. These couples also shared more of their bacteria with each other. In other words, having a dog brought them closer together microbially but having a child did not. The dogs were a conduit shaping the microbiomes of those couples.

In a study from Jack's lab, a family showed a similar influence on microbiome transfer with an outdoor cat.[9] There has been no real test to determine if indoor versus outdoor cats differ in their influence. But we do know that indoor cats are unlikely to have as big a stimulatory influence on the immune system. However, just having any animal around will increase your child's repertoire of microbial exposure.

This all makes sense when you think about it. Our ancestors who domesticated dogs held an advantage over those who didn't bring the animals into their lives. We theorize that people who regularly interacted with dogs developed immune systems that were adapted to canine bacteria. Quite simply, we got used to them. It may be that we are primed to encounter dog bacteria, and when we don't, it's possible that—in some people—the result is an immune malfunction. We don't have a time machine to prove this, but we have plenty of good evidence from animal studies and observations of humans to support this hypothesis.

How dangerous are hospitals? If my child needs surgery, should I worry about hospital-acquired infection? Are all hospitals crawling with superbugs?

No, all hospitals are not crawling with superbugs, and yes, it is safe for your child to go into the hospital.

Remember, hospitals are not inherently dangerous. Hospital staff practically live in them all the time without ever catching a dangerous infection. However, that doesn't stop people from developing life-threatening infections in a hospital. We are all too aware of this. Jack's son has been hospitalized for a broken bone and a few surgeries. And of course, like any parent, Jack has run through the nightmare scenarios in his mind. He does this despite all the evidence he has that his son's chances of infection are extremely small. This is a natural response. Every time Dylan has had to go under general anesthetic, and Jack has had to sign that form that tells the doctors that he understands the risks (which include death), he forgets all of his training and logic, and he panics—if only for a second. Again this is natural: we all do it.

As a professor of surgery Jack works alongside surgeons and has heard many stories and seen many instances where patients have been infected and the surgeons blame themselves. However, more and more evidence suggests that many infections are not the surgeon's fault. Rather, the problem can be traced to a lack of understanding of what happens during surgery.

For example, let's look at gastrointestinal surgery. Since the dawn of surgical practice, the surgeon has understood that gut microbes could influence whether their patient gets better or dies. Mostly this has involved preventing intestinal bacteria from escaping their confines and getting into the body, causing an infection. This, of course, is something to worry about. But on the whole, once prevented, and with the use of antibiotics, a surgeon generally ignores all the surrounding microbes and focuses on fixing the broken human tissue. Then, when an infection occurs, the surgeons and everyone else generally assume they had done something wrong—introduced a bug or missed a stitch.

Only now we realize that the gut microbiome can get very stressed out by surgery itself. The oxygen that leaks in when the gut is cut open is toxic to many of the bacteria that live in there. Then the body is flooded with antibiotics. And finally the body, in trying to repair itself and in responding to its own rather stressful experience, starts to remove phosphate (an important molecule that feeds bacteria) from the gut. This final insult starves the already stressed bacteria, and some of them start to invoke strategies to get the food back—in this case they migrate to the part of the gut that was recently stitched up and proceed to eat the wall.[10] This has catastrophic effects on the human.

So we are just now realizing that a more complete understanding of how bacteria in the gut are affected by surgery is going to be extremely important if we are to prevent postsurgical infections from happening.

If your doctor recommends surgery for your child, you need to evaluate the risks of doing it versus not doing it. This includes direct surgical risks as well as the effects of antibiotics on your child's microbiome. Hospital-acquired infections kill tens of thousands of people each year. On any given day, about one in twenty-five patients will contract an infection. In many cases they may have been carrying the responsible organisms in their bodies when they came in, and the stress of the hospitalization allowed that organism to take over or activate a survival strategy for the bacterium, as highlighted above. Of course there are instances when patients will pick up an infection in the hospital because they are already susceptible and they are exposed either through another infected patient, a surface, or a contaminated instrument—such things do happen. But hospitals have become extremely good at preventing these types of infections. That infections still occur suggests that maybe we need to rethink our strategy, and maybe we need to start treating the patient *and* their microbiome.

Meanwhile, fewer infants are acquiring infections related to their hospital care thanks to a concerted national effort to change the culture in neonatal intensive care units. Doctors, nurses, and staff have redoubled their efforts to keep things clean. For example, they wash their hands more often, remove rings or other wearable items in contact with the outside world, and attend to procedures with renewed vigilance. As a result, between 2007 and 2012 the rates of bloodstream infections from central lines and pneumonia associated with ventilators fell by more than 50 percent.

Is eating dirt really good for my kids?

We've already talked about the hygiene hypothesis. Exposure to farm animals and a wide variety of plants can reduce the risk of atopy, the tendency to allergic sneezing, food allergies, asthma, and skin allergies (atopic dermatitis). So get out and visit some farms if you can and don't worry about germs in the city subways.

But we have another recommendation that parents can pretty much follow anywhere, in the countryside, the suburbs, or city parks. Let your kid play in (and even eat) dirt. Soil is a microbial heaven, with more than a billion bacterial cells per gram, and many fungi and viruses as well. Unless there's lots of animal poop around the soil (which would be a bit gross), you can relax in knowing the soil contains very few organisms that could make your child sick. It is a great source and a great opportunity to expose children to a complex microbial community that will help train their immune system.

Of course there is always the possibility that if your child is immune-compromised or extremely run-down and feeling unwell, there might be bacteria in the soil that could take advantage of his weakened state and make him sicker. But this is still unlikely.

A recent study in the journal *Pediatrics* says that there's some benefit to children putting their grubby little fingers into their mouths.[11] Researchers in New Zealand followed about a thousand people born in 1972–1973 until they were thirty-eight years old. When they were five, seven, nine, and eleven, the research team asked parents if the kids sucked their thumbs or bit their nails. Then they were tested at age thirteen for common allergies to dogs, cats, mold, dust, or grass: 38 percent of those with "oral habits" tested positive, compared to 49 percent of those who kept their hands out of their mouths. This study only points to a correlation, not causation, between these behaviors, but it is nevertheless intriguing.

Thumb-sucking and nail-biting (onychophagia) are nifty ways to deliver dirt. Fingernails are home to 150 or more bacterial species, most flourishing under the nail bed, along with regular dirt. Kids are notorious for getting their hands dirty, so thumbs are an excellent delivery system.

Am I keeping my house too clean? Too dirty? How often should I clean the bathroom?

It's hard to know how clean you should keep your house. Obviously, harmful bacteria such as those from raw chicken or from the surface of unwashed produce need to be kept under control. And you don't want your bathroom to be a den of filth and decomposing feces. It would end up smelling and looking really gross.

However, excessive cleanliness has been linked to a range of conditions, including asthma and allergies, whereas kids who live in households with more diverse microbial communities tend to have lower rates of these diseases.

Some examples of too clean versus too dirty are dealt with

in some of the more specific questions. But here are a few rules to live by. Jack's mother always used to say that a home should be clean enough to be healthy but dirty enough to be happy. No one wants to live in a hospital or a museum. A house should always be lived in, vibrant, and a place of warmth and comfort. First, you only need to steam-clean your carpets if there is an unsightly stain or a bad smell (such as one made by a pet). Regular steam-cleaning for the purpose of "keeping the carpet free of bacteria and other pests" is just nonsense and totally unnecessary.

Consider washing your dishes by hand. Cleaning your dishes in hot water doesn't kill bacteria, but this is a good thing. Households that wash dishes by hand have fewer allergies and less asthma when compared to households that solely use a dishwasher. Give your house a good airing as regularly as possible. This is like spring-cleaning. Get the dust out. That dust is mostly your skin flakes and bacteria from your skin. Opening a window and allowing your house to breathe is a great idea. Get in some houseplants and maybe a pet or two. These are valuable sources of bacteria that can diversify the microbial experience your home provides.

While bleach products may be a good way of getting rid of molds and stains, use them sparingly. You do not need to bleach everything. If you are worried about dangerous food-borne illnesses spread over your kitchen counter, feel free to use an alcohol wipe or hot soapy water to clean the counter—you don't need to bleach it. Mind you, there have been many times Jack has been in a radio interview on the phone giving the same advice, and he will turn around to find his wife doing just that. It's a lesson in humility for him.

For your air conditioner, consider turning it off once in a while and using natural ventilation. This practice saves energy (as long as it is not too hot outside), and it makes you open those windows to exchange the indoor air for outdoor air. Also, regarding air filters in the house, you do not need the $9.99 superfine ultra-grade filters. Get the cheapest ones possible. You won't be hurting your family by doing this. In fact, the cheap ones are designed to stop large particles, which is what the air filters were meant to do in the first place—to keep the air ducts clean.

Live sensibly, apply common sense. Don't live like a germaphobe and you will be fine.

Should I make my toddler wash his hands frequently? How often?

Washing with soap and water is a good idea if your toddler has been touching something likely to have pathogens—say, after visiting a hospital or touching a countertop where raw meat was prepared.

You needn't bother with antibacterial or antiseptic wipes since their benefits are generally overblown. Even alcohol wipes, which are preferable to the antimicrobial brands, can cause issues: the alcohol can dry out your child's hands, making it easier for bad bacteria to colonize them.

Bottom line: hand washing before eating is a good routine to get your toddler into and will greatly reduce the risk of a range of food-borne, fecal-oral, and respiratory diseases. Indeed, according to the Centers for Disease Control and Prevention good hygiene can prevent about 30 percent of diarrhea-related illnesses and 20 percent of colds.

Should I use antibacterial soaps? Hand sanitizers?

No, unless you are working in a health-care setting where more pathogens might be present. For everyday life, soap and water are just fine for keeping your hands clean and your body safe.[12]

On September 3, 2016, the Food and Drug Administration issued a final rule on over-the-counter antibacterial soaps and washes. Moving forward, companies will no longer be allowed to market these products if they contain one or more of nineteen specific active ingredients, including triclosan—a chemical compound that binds to bacterial enzymes and prevents them from reproducing. It has long been added to an enormous number of consumer products, including soaps, hand sanitizers, and body washes (from which it must now be removed), as well as deodorants, detergents, cosmetics, and toothpastes, clothes, kitchenware, furniture, toys, and plastics (where is can still be used.). Triclosan was meant to make products safer by removing "harmful" germs, but as we now know, that's not a great idea because you get rid of the good germs too. (You can't sterilize your way into a longer life.)

Evidence shows that triclosan may harm your child's health. It's an endocrine disruptor that interferes with hormone functions, and there is some evidence that it might disturb thyroid, testosterone, and estrogen regulation, although that evidence is not as strong as some might have you believe. It may disrupt the harmless microbes that colonize your child's body and promote obesity, inflammatory bowel disease, and other behavioral and metabolic disorders. The chemical has also been associated with impaired learning and memory, and it could exacerbate allergies and weaken muscle function; but again the evidence for these claims is not very compelling. It's also been associated with preterm birth and low birth weight. And prolonged exposure during fetal development, infancy, and childhood may lead to permanent damage.

Recently, triclosan gained notoriety when scientists showed

Recently, a handful of studies have started exploring triclosan's impact on the microbiome. One found that antibacterial soaps are no more effective in removing bacteria than regular soap and water. The study went on to show that the only way that triclosan-containing soap could outperform regular soap was by applying it for nine hours. And who washes their hands for nine hours?

Another fed high doses of triclosan to zebra fish (a common laboratory organism as well as a mainstay of the inexpensive sections at pet stores) over the course of a week. The researchers observed shifts in the structure, diversity, and interaction networks of the fish's microbiome as well as an increase in bacteria resistant to triclosan. But fish exposed for only four days did not show such changes.

A third study added low, environmentally relevant doses of triclosan to the habitat of fathead minnows. After one week, the fish exhibited changes in gut microbe diversity. But after two weeks with no exposure to triclosan, their microbiome had returned to its original composition and structure.

Finally, a study published in 2016 studied triclosan's effect on the microbes living with us humans. They compared volunteers who used personal products (toothpaste, hand and liquid soap, and dish soap) with and without triclosan for four months at a time. All volunteers in contact with triclosan had higher concentrations of it in their urine but showed no changes in their stool or oral microbiomes. Also, there were no changes in their hormone levels.[13]

We can think of a few possible explanations for the disparities between these studies. The zebra fish and minnows were exposed to far more triclosan than the people were. We also tend to immediately rinse off products like toothpaste and soap. Another possibility is that triclosan exposure is

that bacteria can become insensitive or resistant to it, which was often reported as helping give rise to antibiotic-resistant superbugs. But this concern is not really accurate. Although bacteria may become resistant to triclosan, it is not used as a clinical antibiotic. There's simply no evidence that resistance to triclosan could induce resistance to the antibiotics your doctor prescribes.

Triclosan has made its way into the bodies of 75 percent of the U.S. population. Tests find it in blood, urine, and breast milk. Alarmed, the European Union banned products containing triclosan in 2010. The state of Minnesota did the same two years later. In 2013, the Food and Drug Administration issued a rule requiring manufacturers of antibacterial consumer goods to prove that their products are safe by September 2016. As a result, Procter & Gamble immediately eliminated triclosan from many of its products.

But there are other options. Alcohol-based hand sanitizers do not contain triclosan. So if you ever feel the need to wipe germs off your hands, you have an excellent alternative. Nevertheless, the evidence for or against this type of hand sanitizer is surprisingly weak. Alcohol-based hand sanitizers have been shown to kill a lot of harmful germs, so if you're exposed to someone who's sick or visiting a clinic or hospital where sick kids congregate, you should probably use the products there. But repeated and unnecessary use of hand sanitizers may deplete the natural protective microbial community on your skin. This may make it easier for the bad bugs to colonize you and then get passed on to your baby. So just like other antimicrobials, you want to limit hand sanitizers to the situations where you think there are real risks.

so ubiquitous, even starting in the womb, that our microbes have already adapted to the chemical. People who did not come into contact with triclosan over the four-month period still had detectable levels of it in their urine, although unsurprisingly at lower concentrations.

More research is needed to determine if triclosan affects human microbial communities at all. We don't know, for example, if metabolic by-products of triclosan affect the structure of our gut microbes. We need to look at dose, timing, and route of triclosan exposure. Triclosan is readily absorbed through our skin and GI tract, but we tend to apply it topically, unlike the fish who ate it. Our exposures are small and transient when using personal care products such as toothpaste. But the triclosan found in surface, ground, and drinking water raises the risk that it might accumulate in our tissues.

Finally, if effects of triclosan are observed in our guts, are these changes reversible? Are there key developmental windows during which microbiome perturbations can leave lasting impacts on neurological and immune development? If so, even short, low-concentration exposures to triclosan may alter the gut flora and health of developing infants, so prenatal, perinatal, and postnatal triclosan exposure may be more detrimental than adult exposure.

Can you provide a few guiding principles for how to choose baby products such as antifungal rash cream, antibiotic wipes, and the like?

In general, most baby products have been tested for what they do for the particular condition they're designed to get rid of, but not for what side effects they might have on your baby's microbiome in the longer term. Be aware that any product that doesn't fall under FDA regulation may have no scientific evidence backing it. However, that doesn't necessarily mean that it doesn't work. Also, just because there has not been a study to show whether a product is safe doesn't mean it is safe. The fact that we do not know just means that it hasn't been worthwhile for anyone to do a test.

However, many of the products you can buy do have listed side effects, and unless we are talking about a medicine that your child needs, then you might want to think again before using them. For example, antibacterial wipes may seem like a good idea, but if they contain triclosan you might consider using an alcohol-based wipe. Of course these can dry out your baby's skin.

A better alternative might be a gentle brand of soap and water, which are effective in eliminating harmful bacteria and viruses. So if your kid just picked up something truly disgusting off the floor, don't worry. Grab the soap and water and scrub your child's hands vigorously for at least twenty seconds. (The CDC recommends singing the "Happy Birthday" song twice, which you can do with a clear conscience since it's out of copyright.) Researchers working in Rob's microbiology lab at UC San Diego are taught to use soap and water in their safety training.

One thing for sure, it's not easy to know what products to trust. Anyone with two children, like Jack, will know that you are way more careful and cautious with what your first child is exposed to. Once you get the hang of it, the second child is not given as much cotton-wool protection. With his first child, he and his wife used cloth diapers and natural water wipes with no chemicals. When Dylan got a fungal infection or diaper rash, they ended up using probiotic yogurt to cure the infection. Would he recommend that you do this with your child? Possibly. But by the time his second child arrived, they were back in disposable diapers, using whatever wipes they could lay their hands on at the time, and Hayden never got a fungal infection. So each child is different. We cannot therefore recommend a specific way of doing things, but instead suggest that you trust your instincts and be inquisitive as to what is in a particular product.

Is it okay for my child to touch poop?

The delight of having your child touch poop, or even eat it, is familiar to many parents. How much you should panic depends on whose poop it is. If it's your child's own poop, or a family member's, the good news is that they are probably already exposed to those microbes. So it's gross, but in the grand scheme of things it doesn't matter that much. If it's outside the family, you still don't have to worry as long as no pathogens are present. Fact is, the world is covered in a fine patina of feces, spread from people's hands or degraded and spread into the air. In the end we are all made from molecules that were once poop, maybe a dinosaur's poop. Tell that to the kids.

For dog poop, most canine microbes don't colonize the human gut and vice versa, so your kid is probably fine. However, some parasites and illnesses can be transmitted across species, including giardia, cryptosporidium, and worms of various kinds, fungi, and bacteria, including *Salmonella* and *Campylobacter*. If you keep your dog healthy and poop is consumed, don't worry.

The biggest risk is touching feces from sick people. If your kid isn't a poop glutton and there's some left over, you might want to save it and get it tested at a hospital for a stool-borne and blood-borne pathogen panel (keep it frozen). However, the general poison control advice is that stool is considered "minimally toxic" (even if it's maximally disgusting), and most of the bacterial effects happen in four to eight hours. So unless you have a specific reason to think the person or animal that produced the stool is ill, your best bet is to watch your kid at home and only take him to the hospital if there's vomiting or diarrhea.

When should I expose my infant to strangers?

A common guideline is six to eight weeks. The reason is that your newborn's immune system is still developing, and strangers could carry a disease that they may not disclose, which could threaten your child's health.

As we mentioned elsewhere, the chances of a stranger's microbiome harming your child are extremely low. It's even possible that his or her nonpathogen microbiome could be beneficial. But you have to weigh the risks. If the stranger is some random woman on a bus who fusses over your baby, perhaps pull back. But if the stranger is someone you meet at a friend's house, it's probably safe to hand her your baby.

At the earliest ages, your newborn's behavioral responses are limited, so if he gets an infection you might not know there's a problem until it's too late. Symptoms are typically vague, including irritability, problems feeding, irregular breathing, crying, and other things babies do all the time. They may not get a fever even in the face of a severe infection. So if you take your baby out earlier, monitor them carefully for signs of problems, and keep in mind that these signals may be very subtle.

Is my child picking up bad microbes from friends at school? What about foreign students at our preschool?

Your child is almost certainly exchanging microorganisms with the other children and school staff. Whether she is getting more good than bad microbes is still a matter of controversy. It's every parent's experience, including our own, that preschools can resemble cesspools of infectious disease. Kids come home with colds, flu, chicken pox, mysterious rashes, lice, and other unsavory hitchhikers. With the speed of a toddler racing down a hall, these maladies can spread to other family members.

Jack recalls the first time his kids got lice at school. He was in India at a conference and his wife, Kat, was frantic. He felt for her from a distance as she boiled clothes, sterilized the entire house, and applied all kind of shampoos and combs to remove the nits, or lice eggs. When he finally got home after a very long, and tiring flight, he was asked to strip as soon as he walked in the door. All his clothes were boiled and he, too, had to wash in antilice shampoo. He was very perplexed by this level of sanitation, as he had not been in the house when the outbreak occurred. But Kat was adamant that it had to be done. So being very jet-lagged he just went along with it.

Overall, though, Jack's family rarely gets acute diseases that appear to come from school, possibly helped by the fact that their elementary school has very strict rules about kids showing up with illness. For example, if a child says she feels hot, a phone call goes out to a parent to have the child isolated and removed. Jack is sure that more than once his kids have used this policy as a stratagem to get a day off from school.

But are these microepidemics all bad? We've been arguing that you want to expose your little ones to the widest possible diversity of microbes, good and bad—but not so bad that they threaten long-term health. There's a huge difference in terms of immune development between catching the common cold and coming down with hepatitis.

Contact with contagious disease is inevitable in school settings, so we recommend you don't fret about it. Most infections are self-limited, and you have access to advanced medical care if you need it. If you worry that kids from foreign countries may bring exotic diseases into school, don't. U.S. immigration policy requires proof of vaccination for children entering the country. Also, importantly, unless a child is overtly sick, the possibility that he or she will be contagious with a major infection is extremely low.

In terms of a rich, diverse microbial exposure, if your children are exposed to a foreign child for a prolonged period of time, this could actually help improve their microbial diversity, which could have unforeseen health benefits. And you never know: they might learn a new language as well.

Do I bring home bad microbes from work?

Each person sheds 38 million microbes an hour, so every time you interact with people you are picking up some of their germs.[14] So you certainly bring microbes home from work, as well as from every other environment that you go to. But whether these germs are bad is another question. Unless you work somewhere that has nasty pathogens, like a morgue or a hospital, you're probably fine. However, if you do work in one of those places, you definitely want to wash your hands carefully and, if necessary, use sanitizer before interacting with your family.

Jack has worked in and around microbiological laboratories for his entire career, and this potential source of dangerous organisms was never a concern until his first child arrived. Then his wife worried that one of the microbial strains he was working with might hitch a ride into their home. If the microbes ever did, they never caused any problems. But it did make Jack wonder how others view people like him who sometimes wear green medical scrubs outside of the hospital. There's a perception that scrubs must be covered in those dangerous superbugs that everyone is always talking about. Hospitals are dangerous places right? Well, yes, but it's extraordinarily unlikely that a nurse would be wearing a scrub infected with a lethal agent that could be transmitted in public and make anyone sick.

The truth is, hospitals, laboratories, and places such as meat-processing plants, where potentially dangerous organisms might hang around, all have extremely stringent safety guidelines that staff need to adhere to, for their own safety as much as anyone else's.

People often ask us if a stranger's bacteria could be bad for their child. We've been telling you that bacteria are moving about quite freely between most of us—should you let outsiders near their children? It makes sense that you may fear "dirty" people at work may have "contaminated" you with their own breed of "dirty" microbes. But please remember, the bacteria on human beings are all very, very similar. In fact, while we can identify individuals by the strains of bacteria they carry (leading to a field of microbial forensics, which both Jack and Rob are very interested in), we can still tell if the microbes on your skin are human microbes, especially when we compare them with the microbes on a dog, a monkey, or a fish. So don't fret about strangers' bacteria. They're mostly the same general kinds of bacteria that you carry around.

This realization is how Jack lost his disgust for public restrooms. All those bodily secretions from other people seemed utterly gross. He hated them. The smell alone made him picture the kind of person he didn't want to picture, doing the kinds of things he didn't want to know about. But in our modern world, where most major transmissible diseases have been eradicated, it's extremely unlikely that he (or you) would encounter anything—microbially speaking—dangerous in a bathroom. In the end, all he saw was just another bathroom load of human skin bacteria.[15]

Rob, working with collaborators at the University of Colorado, looked at all the sources of bacteria in dormitory restroom stalls. The sampling proceeded mostly without incident. They went early in the morning to collect samples, making sure the restrooms were unoccupied before and during their tasks. Naturally when the bathrooms were locked, some students were not happy. One day a note was taped to the door saying "Girls, stay out of the boys' bathroom!"

The researchers found that fecal bacteria were primarily confined to the stall itself, and what you see on the toilet seat is human skin bacteria. When public toilets do become foul (and we've all experienced that), the mess can be cleaned up to restore the bathroom to resemble any old bathroom. This fact doesn't stop Jack from getting annoyed that some people seem incapable of using bathrooms without making them dirty. But case in point, if he sees a used paper towel on the floor, he is highly likely to pick it up and put it in the trash.

My toddler ate something off the floor. Should I worry? How long should I wait before taking it away from her?

The five-second rule states that food or cutlery dropped on the ground will not be significantly contaminated with bacteria if you pick it up within five seconds of its being dropped. This may sound appealing, but it's not true.[16] As soon as food, a spoon, a pacifier, or grubby little fingers touch a surface before going into your child's mouth, the objects will pick up bacterial cells present on that surface. If that surface is moist or sticky, for example, a piece of toast covered in butter or jam, then it is probable that more cells will be picked up.

But what's the issue here? Should you always forbid your kids to pop items into their mouths that they've picked up from the floor? Is a yuck factor at play? Should you worry about potential exposure to pathogens?

Much depends on what they pick up from the floor and the nature of that floor. Obviously, if your child nabs a piece of rotting food, you'll want to get it out of her hands and mouth as soon as possible and then monitor her for infection. This doesn't mean she will get sick, but she's more likely to get sick from that than from picking up and mouthing a toy truck (though she could choke on it). If your baby picks up an item from your living room floor, you'll know more or less how clean it is. If the surface is a filthy alley, maybe not so much. Use your judgment.

Babies train their immune systems one mouthful of microbes after another. In fact it is possible that the reflex babies seem to have for putting things into their mouths may have evolved to increase their early microbial exposure. Of course we have no evidence of this, but it is a theory that would fit the available evidence.

Should I sterilize my baby's pacifier? Should I lick it?

There's no credible evidence that the practice of licking your infant's pacifier poses any danger whatsoever. Just the opposite.[17] Swedish scientists looked at the pacifier-cleaning practices of 184 babies and their parents. About half the parents said they rinsed the pacifier in water and occasionally boiled it. The other half said they sucked the pacifier clean before giving it back to their babies.

By the time the babies were eighteen months old, those whose parents "cleaned" their pacifier by sucking it were less likely to have asthma, eczema, or sensitivity to food and airborne allergens. Microbes in the parent's saliva evidently stimulated the baby's immune system to help ward off those conditions.

There are dentists out there who caution that this practice could transmit bacteria or viruses from you to your baby. So if you have poor dental hygiene, gum disease or bleeding gums, cold sores, canker sores, a sore throat, or some other problem with your mouth and throat, just don't do it. But if you're healthy, there's no evidence that swapping saliva, eating from the same bowl, or licking a pacifier poses a danger to your baby.

Don't be paranoid. You want to put friendly microbes into your baby.

I heard that the New York City subway carries microbes that cause plague and anthrax. Is it safe for me to take my child down into the subway?

It's safe and here's why. Efforts are under way to assess microbes in the "built environment," meaning homes, office buildings, hospitals, and other public spaces. We have discussed some of this in sections on air-conditioning, household cleanliness, washing dishes, and so on. But the long and the short of it is this: the built environment mostly contains dead bacteria from humans that are shed from our bodies and die in the inhospitable desert that is a concrete slab, a dry carpet, a table top, or a tiled floor. Without moisture, nutrients, or a host to call home, these bugs usually expire. Those that don't die immediately could be transferred between people, but it's extremely rare to find them in high enough numbers on a surface that they could be contagious. An exception is a sickroom where a person suffers from a communicable disease. But most sickrooms are isolated from the outside world. You're not going to enter many of them in your lifetime unless you're a health-care provider, and health-care providers know how to protect themselves.

However, a recent study found evidence of plague and anthrax in the New York subway.[18] Only the study was wrong. A subsequent reanalysis of the data, as well as a new study of the Boston subway, found no pathogens—only skin microbes, most of which were likely dead and environmental generalists.[19] The subways are as safe as your living room. In fact, there were even fewer antibiotic-resistant microbes in the subway than in the gut of an average human. All bacterial communities have antibiotic resistance, as they have to fight other bacteria that are trying to kill them with their own arsenals of microbial antibiotics. The subway was virtually devoid of these, though, probably because most bacteria were dead.

Here's the problem. When we analyze DNA isolated from an environment, we characterize each unknown microbial community by comparing its DNA sequences to databases of known DNA sequences (remember that microbes have their own DNA, so we're not talking here about human DNA left in the environment). However, in most cases, microbial life is quite diverse, so a lot of the DNA sequences we come across, while they may have some similarity to a known piece of DNA in the database, might be something completely different. But reporting an unknown is not very exciting, so sometimes researchers can get carried away trying to find a "story" in their data. Luckily, in nearly all cases of this, the scientific community rises up if they cannot reproduce the findings and calls them out.

One of Rob's favorite examples comes from using sequencing data to detect *Salmonella* in fresh produce.[20] There was no evidence of the pathogen in the tomato crop, but samples collected from the roots and leaves found the surprising presence of red jungle fowl, house mouse, and the elusive duck-billed platypus. Hey, there's false evidence of platypus genes in the human gut, too. Of course there is no duck-billed platypus on the leaves of a tomato plant or in the human gut (unless you ate one of course), but if researchers are desperate enough to want to name every piece of DNA they find, they could report that this is what they found. Which of course would be wrong.

Hence, don't believe everything you read. This is an important reason why we wrote this book. There is a lot of information out there, and we wanted to distill it down so that what you read here is the reliable evidence made accessible.

Should my child take communion?

This decision will probably be made within each family based on factors other than the strictly scientific. However, from a microbiome perspective, highly processed carbohydrates such as those used in the wafers aren't very good for your child. Alcohol in small doses is good for microbial diversity but has not been looked at in young children. As you can imagine, it would be hard to get funding for such a study or to get people to sign their babies or toddlers up for it.

On the other hand, shared drinking vessels can transmit colds and flu as well as more serious pathogens such as tuberculosis. This is why a major campaign to replace "the common cup" with drinking fountains was conducted in the early twentieth century, with admirable public health benefits.

On the whole it is unlikely that your child will catch anything from taking communion, and we have no evidence as to whether the exposure to other people's oral microbiome could improve or impact her health.

Should I wash dishes in the dishwasher or by hand? What's best for microbial health?

You may be surprised to learn that hand-washing beats dish-washers.[21] The reason relates to our old friend the hygiene hypothesis. Many older dishwashers use a heating cycle to dry the dishes after the wash cycle, which actively kills most bacteria. You want your kid to be exposed to more, not fewer, bacteria in daily life.

By comparison, washing dishes by hand in warm water doesn't kill bacteria. It just washes off the visible food residue. This means hand-washed dishes have more microbes, which may help to train and stimulate your child's immune system. A study carried out in two Swedish towns found that dishwashing by hand was associated with a reduced risk of children developing allergies. However, the study did not prove whether hand-washing dishes caused the reduced risk of allergies, because both of these could be driven by some other factor in the same households.

To determine whether machine dishwashing reduces microbial exposure and thereby increases allergies, we would have to intervene in people's lives. Some would be allowed to use a dishwasher, while others would not. Ideally we would do this without them knowing we were doing it, and we would do this for thousands of people. Not only would this be virtually impossible to do, it would also be prohibitively expensive. This is an ideal example of why we don't always have the answers. And why we often have to rely on correlative studies.

Another issue is that as a way of saving energy newer dishwashers don't use a heating cycle. Instead they use chemicals that stop water from pooling on the dishes as they dry. We have no idea what these chemicals do to bacteria, but they may make dishes too dry, which will also kill a lot of bacteria.

Jack recently purchased one of these new no-heat-cycle dishwashers, and while he is excited about the potential energy-saving benefits, he's also slightly concerned about the rinse aid used to dry the dishes. Rinse aid causes water to form small droplets, which then evaporate or run off the plates and cutlery more easily. Many of these chemicals in high concentrations do have known side effects; you should never drink rinse aid, for example. We have no evidence that rinse aid is damaging for your microbiome, especially after having been through the dishwasher. But Jack is keeping a close eye on the literature. It is convenient, but at the first sign of trouble, he and his kids will be doing the dishes by hand.

How often should I bathe my child?

No specific research from a microbiome perspective has been done on how frequently your child should bathe. Even in atopic dermatitis, a skin condition linked to the immune system and microbiome, there are no consistent recommendations from health authorities on the best bathing frequency and duration.

One study suggests that children who bathe more frequently are more likely to get asthma.[22] But we could not find any epidemiological evidence linking bathing frequency in young children to asthma, allergies, or other diseases of the microbiome, which is interesting given the intense interest recently in the hygiene hypothesis.

A lot of municipal water in the United States is highly chlorinated, which is one reason why you feel so sleepy in a hot bath. The hot water liberates the chlorine, which you inhale, causing a sedative effect. There is a possibility that this could damage the microbiome on your baby's skin. But we should stress that there have been no studies to test whether this actually happens.

Jack's children love baths and will spend inordinate amounts of time wallowing in the warm water. Neither of them have any skin conditions of note. He and his wife also love baths as a nice way of isolating themselves for a while. They considered getting one of those municipal water-conditioning systems for their home to dechlorinate and "clean up" their water chemistry, but in the end they didn't do it. Jack can't say that anyone in his family has had any side effects from excessive bathing.

Rob's daughter also loves the water, whether it's a bath, a swimming pool, or the ocean. He hasn't made any effort to avoid exposing her to chlorine, although it's something he worries about from time to time. They do have a water filter in their fridge, though the parents don't stop her from drinking tap water if it's more convenient.

Should I let my child drink from a public water fountain? Should I give my child tap water or bottled water?

To the best of our knowledge there are no risks in drinking from a public water fountain in the developed world. But there are risks associated with both city water and bottled water.

We've already talked about bisphenol A—BPA—which can have implications for the development of children, including their microbiome. And while this compound has been removed from a lot of plastics, it can still be found in many plastic bottles. So that would be a potential risk for bottled water.

As for public water fountains, a lot of city water has high levels of chlorine and other minerals that could negatively influence your child's microbiome. However, we should stress that you would have to drink extraordinary quantities of city water (except in a few specific locations such as Hong Kong) to cause this problem.

On the whole, Jack and Rob have no problem with their kids drinking from either water fountains or water bottles. They actively do both. Despite potential risks, the dangers of dehydration are significantly higher.

My child touched a snake. Do snakes carry dangerous bacteria?

Jack and Rob both grew up with captive snakes. To the best of our knowledge neither of us ever got sick from touching one. At age six, Jack joined the Young Herpetologists (part of the British Herpetological Society) where he engaged his passion for finding out as much as possible about the best way to keep reptiles and amphibians, including what they ate, what kind of environment they liked, and even how to keep them entertained. It was always important to him to make sure the animals were kept happy. Remember, this was the time before Google, so he had to get his information mainly from the library or society newsletters. He mostly kept garter snakes and finds it interesting that garter snakes thrive in the wild around his house. In Illinois, they are often sunbathing on the prairie paths, and it is always fun to catch them to show to the kids—and then let them go free.

Six years ago, Rob published paper on the postprandial remodeling of the gut microbiota in Burmese pythons.[23] These magnificent animals are sit-and-wait foragers that consume large prey at long intervals. Rob wanted to know how their guts manage it. When a python eats a large animal, it's basically performing a heroic athletic feat, and its internal organs, like its heart and liver, radically transform themselves, increasing in mass by 30 to 40 percent. He wanted to see if the same was true for the microbiome. During fasting, the python's gut shrinks to a vanishingly small size, and its microbiome transforms into a state with more bacteria that feed off cell walls, but very low total amounts of bacteria. When a python swallows a rat, its microbiome is completely reshaped, with a lot more fast-growing bacteria like Firmicutes. Their community resembles that of a fat mouse (which we know from other studies), suggesting that different species' microbiomes may respond the same way to extreme diet. One thing he and his colleagues had to check was whether the microbes were coming in via the rat. To find this out they had to sample the rat the way the snake does, that is, the whole rat. So they bought an industrial-strength blender to grind up the whole rat and sample all its microbes. This let them show that most of the microbes were from the snake, growing as fast as they could once they had a rat to digest.

However, snakes, other reptiles, and birds can harbor strains of *Salmonella*. We know of instances where infants became infected after drinking water visited by a snake. Of course, your chances of being infected are greater if you handle the animal directly. This is common sense. You should always wash your hands after handling any wild animal because they can harbor dangerous pathogens (think Ebola, salmonellosis, and influenza) that can be transmitted to humans.

Therefore, if your children have snakes or have the possibility of being in contact with snakes, keep an eye on them if they get diarrhea. Tell your doctor they may have been exposed to *Salmonella*.

At the same time, it's possible that exposure to animal microbiomes could help train your child's immune system and help prevent immune-related diseases. However, we stress that we have no evidence for this—just a love of snakes.

What does travel do to my child's microbiome?

Most of what we know about how travel affects the microbiome comes from studies of adults, so it may not apply to children. This is because children are vulnerable and research involving them comes under especially tough ethical scrutiny. Unless the research is specifically about kids, we tend to carry out early studies on adult volunteers. Nevertheless, the way in which microbes interact with one another and interact with the human body has many commonalities across age. And especially when it comes to travel, the trends we have observed in children fit our predictions based on the microbial evidence from adults.

All life on Earth is dictated by daily fluctuations of light caused by the planet's rotation around its axis. This phenomenon gave rise to a number of biological clocks—oscillators that anticipate and keep track of time in organisms as environmental conditions change. All creatures have biological clocks, from the tiniest microbes to the great blue whales.

As for humans, your body has a master clock in your brain but also dozens of clocks in various organs, tissues, and other parts of your body that control metabolism, behavior, and immunity. They all need to be synchronized for you to feel and stay healthy.

Your gut microbes also show diurnal shifts, though not to light. They respond to food and the timing of meals. Depending on your habits, different species flourish at different times of day and release different metabolites. These molecules act on circadian clock genes in your liver, synchronizing metabolism with the rest of your body. And here is where jet lag comes in.

When you travel through several time zones, your central and peripheral clocks become disconnected and fall out of equilibrium. This is because your eyes, which are the portals into your central circadian rhythms in your brain, are sensing a different time. But the clocks in your other organs (liver, kidneys, gut, etc.) have not yet gotten the message, so they continue to function as if you were awake when you are sleeping, and as if you are asleep when you are awake. This causes jet lag. Children and adults both suffer from the same phenomenon.

Recent research has shown that your gut microbes don't adjust as quickly as your brain does to the new time zone.[24] Their rhythms are likely coordinated by when food comes in, and by the immune and hormonal signals that are driven by the rest of your body's clocks. So the microbes don't get reset. Their oscillations are now aberrant, and the chemical signals they are sending out cause more mayhem inside your already confused body.

In some studies, these confused chemical signals—especially to the liver—have been implicated in causing the weight gain experienced by night shift workers. If you work those odd hours, or you are constantly changing time zones, you're more likely to put on weight given the same calorific intake.

We know the details of this cascade from animal studies that show jet lag, or circadian rhythm disruption, influences on the gut microbiome. The body is a massively interconnected system, and when you disrupt one thing—as in the sense of time—you will affect other parts of the system.

Similarly, if you eat lots of high-fat, sugary foods, you are likely to disrupt your microbiome's rhythm, and this too can lead to weight gain.[25] A poor diet may tell your liver it's noon when your brain thinks it's morning.

On the other hand, when you're traveling you're probably eating more, especially more junk food. Come on! We all do it, especially when traveling with kids. Each year, Jack and Kat take their boys (and two dogs) on a thousand-mile road trip to Woods Hole, Massachusetts, where Jack works at a laboratory for a month each summer. They tend to do the trip in a grueling seventeen-hour push. Obviously, there's little time to sit down and eat healthy meals, especially not in the kind of restaurants you find on the road. So, yes, the diet plan does slip.

As we have pointed out in other sections—increased sugar intake and fatty foods can lead to an increase in bacteria that may cause inflammation. So during such a trip we may also be causing unintended inflammation. Anecdotally, people often get sores in their mouth or disrupted gastrointestinal activity when they do long drives, and the implication has always been that people eat poor diets or are just sitting for too long. Although the evidence is weak, it could be that these activities also increase pro-inflammatory bacteria, which could cause systemic inflammation far away from your gut, and hence could even result in those mouth sores.

How to combat this? We don't have a scientifically proven way but on our long road trips we follow common sense. We swap candy for fruit and bring plenty of water instead of soda. But occasionally fast-food restaurants are our only choice, so we go with it.

. . . .

An obvious threat to your child's microbiome and to yours while traveling is the possibility of picking up a nasty pathogen. Depending on where you are in the world, it's easy to pick up a bug, especially those that cause diarrhea. Sometimes it is hard to rid these bugs from your gut; or they can cause a long-term shift in your microbial community to a pro-inflammatory state. This is why some people, long after the original infection is gone, still get loose bowel movements and irritable-bowel symptoms.

In many parts of the world, local bacteria can easily infect food and water. Of course you can drink bottled water or soda, avoid street food and fruits without peels, and forgo ice. But one of our colleagues got cholera from eating a watermelon in India. The farmer had injected it with local water to make it heavier, which got him a higher price, but our friend became quite ill.

Jack has only had traveler's diarrhea twice in his life, once when he ate a roasted guinea pig from a street vendor in Cusco, Peru—but that was more likely food poisoning, plain and simple. The second time he was in China, and both he and his wife got diarrhea that stayed with them for a number of weeks, with periods of quiet between bouts of gut cramps and loose stool.

You may be vulnerable to diarrhea for a couple of reasons. When you eat a different diet, your microbiome is disrupted, leaving your gut open to invasion by an opportunistic pathogen. If you encounter one, your whole microbial community is thrown out of balance, and even after the pathogen has been passed or surpassed, the effects of this disruption can sometimes be felt months later.

There's an interesting story from China related to this. When officials used to travel to distant parts of the country, they would always take a small pot of soil from their home with them. When they were in their distant post, and they got traveler's diarrhea, they would take some of the soil, mix it with water, and drink the slurry. This was prescribed as a cure. Maybe there is something to this, although be aware we have no credible evidence. Maybe just experiencing bacteria from the environment in which you grew up, or to which you have become accustomed, could help your gut microbiome to recover against an invading pathogen. Of course virtually none of these soil bacteria could take up residence in your gut, but like many probiotics you buy off the shelf (which also do not take up residence), they may just be what your immune system needs to help fight off an infection. This would be really exciting to test.

Whether the effect of travel is bad overall—because of jet lag, junk food, or the likelihood of picking up Delhi belly or Montezuma's revenge—or good because you and your child are exposed to a wider range of friendly microbes is still unknown.

Of course it may depend on your specific destination. In 2014, Jack and Kat took their boys to China for work. Jack was giving lectures all over the country, but their hosts were kind enough to also show the family around during the visit. One time they all went to Kunming, Yunnan Province. And from there, they went to the Honghe Hanei Rice Terraces—which are truly beautiful. In a small Hanei village, where most people are subsistence farmers living day to day, they found a lady who was willing to cook them some lunch. Much to everyone's surprise, no less the boys, the woman grabbed a chicken off the road, beheaded it, and started to prepare it on a wooden block next to her home. The boys watched with fascination. Jack watched with a mix of fascination and fear—what if we caught some nasty gut bug that made us all sick? He didn't want to spend the next three days on the toilet. However, the woman took the chicken meat, grilled it, and then cooked it with noodles to make a soup. The boys ate it and no one got sick. It was a fascinating cultural experience for the boys but also a good indication that carefully cooked, fresh food, is rarely going to make you sick.

. . . .

One final note: we often get asked about airplanes and how "germy" they are. Once flying, the air on a plane is recirculated, but it is also passed through special filters that can remove viral particles.[26] This filtration happens six times a minute on most planes, for the entire volume of air in the aircraft. So you can be rest assured that the air is very clean.

Of course there's always the possibility that surfaces in the plane could be contaminated with a virus left behind on a seat back. If you touch it and then pick your nose or put your fingers in your mouth, you have an increased probability of getting an infection. It's also likely that the physical stress and disrupted circadian rhythm that many people experience on a plane could throw your whole system into disequilibrium, and so your natural defenses could be down. This could make you susceptible to an infection.

In truth, though, airplanes are no more germy than other places, and if you are in good health, you have nothing to worry about. We each travel more than 150,000 miles a year and we do not see a correlation between travel and getting sick.

I heard that Finnish and Swedish parents let their infants sleep outdoors. Does that improve microbial health? Should I open the windows?

The practice of parents in Nordic countries allowing their infants to nap outside (of course, wrapped up well) stems from the 1940s, when indoor air quality was generally a lot worse than it is now. Kerosene lamps and heaters and wood or coal heating and cooking are known to be bad for infant health because of carbon monoxide, particulates from smoke, and other issues. Fortunately, these have been essentially replaced by electric appliances, so many of the perceived benefits may not be relevant today. No study has directly examined the potential impact of infants sleeping outside, especially since it's hard to come up with a placebo.

One of Rob's postdoctoral researchers, Chris Callewaert, says that his mom always told him that the bedroom temperature should not be too warm. In his family, the bedrooms were never heated. In this society of thermostats and central heating, we are rarely exposed to cold temperatures. This may weaken our immune systems. In Belgium they say: "As weak as a greenhouse plant." A greenhouse plant will not be able to withstand the windy, cold, and rainy environment outside. This may relate to humans. If you're constantly in a warm environment, you are probably more likely to get sick when a virus is around, just because your immune system is 'on low mode.' One study showed that acute cold exposure (men sitting for two hours at 5°C) had an immunostimulatory effect. In other words, being exposed to cold makes your immune system stronger and may help in preventing catching a cold. Chris speaks from experience: he was in boarding school for five years and regularly caught a cold. When somebody in the classroom caught a cold, he could only count the days before he got it as well. After he started riding his bike to school, through the rain, wind, and cold, he almost never caught a cold again.

One thing we know for sure, indoor air quality is frequently an issue. In many developing countries, children suffer from respiratory conditions brought on by being raised in a home with an open fire or stove in an insufficiently ventilated area. The World Health Organization has even said that reducing reliance on indoor wood-burning stoves for heat and cooking is one of the key areas of improvement that would dramatically reduce childhood mortality rates around the world.

However, from the perspective of the microbiome, there is very little data on how indoor air quality specifically influences infant health. We know that damp, musty homes can cause respiratory and allergy problems due to overexposure to mold and fungal spores. Jack dealt with this issue when he and his family lived in England in a 150-year-old granite cottage that used to house the coaches, horses, and coachmen for the manor up the hill. It was lovely, quaint, and unique and they adored it. But there was constant concern over the potential for all that dampness to influence the family's health. Sometimes they could smell the mold. Although Jack and his wife have no evidence that these conditions did or did not influence the boys' health, they were always airing out the house, keeping windows and doors open for long periods, and spending a lot of time walking the kids either around the town or in the nearby countryside. They have a lot of photos on epic treks with the kids in a stroller. It was not easy.

Back in 2011 there was a resurgence of interest in the microbiome of buildings. This continues today, and both Jack and Rob have played significant roles in shaping this field. Working alongside architects and indoor air scientists we have gained a fundamental perspective of the potential risks. Many of them are chemical. Poor air ventilation mixed with dampness, both in homes and preschools, increases the risk that children might develop atopy or lung disease. It is definitely something to look out for.

However, a neglected area was always the indoor bacterial communities and what they looked like. We started to apply genomic sequencing tools to explore the bacteria living in our homes, and what we found was fascinating. Most bacteria in a home come from the skin of the inhabitants, not from dirt blown or tracked in and not from insects, rodents, or other unintended housemates. A seminal study in 2011 demonstrated that opening windows in a hospital could reduce the abundance of potential bacterial pathogens in the facility, recapitulating work that

Florence Nightingale had tested in the mid-nineteenth century.[27] She found that if she let fresh air into a ward, it helped injured soldiers to recover. She didn't necessarily know why, but the practice persists today. The basic premise is that you can get a buildup of bacteria from people in any enclosed indoor space. If you add sick people, the air and surfaces could become rich with disease-causing bacteria. If you open the window, you let in lots of benign bacteria from the outdoors, which swamp the bad bacteria. This significantly reduces the chance that people in the room will encounter the kinds of bacteria that make them sick.

Another important component comes into play. As we have talked about elsewhere, every baby is essentially free of bacteria before birth and is brought into the world with a healthy dose of the mother's bacteria. They then get a dose of bacteria from anyone else who starts to interact with them. In the old days, the baby might have been taken back to a farm or a home with leaky walls and plenty of microbial exposure—so much so that his or her descendants would have immune systems that would be adapted to expect to see all of that rich microbial exposure. Today, a baby is given antibiotics prophylactically at birth and brought back to an overly sterile home, with sealed windows and constantly "conditioned" air, possibly with strong filtration to remove any possible allergens. The child's parents take great care to ensure the house is very clean. Where is the microbial exposure that the child's immune system is expecting? Absent. Instead the infant is exposed to a constant stream of skin-associated bacteria from the parents. Maybe none of these cause disease, but let's face it, if you are expecting soil, tree, cow, pig, chicken, and dog-associated bacteria, and instead you get just more human-skin bacteria, your immune system may not get the interactions it's expecting to function the way it did in the past.

So maybe letting your baby sleep outside—as long as she is

protected from the weather (hot or cold)—will increase her exposure to a diverse array of benign bacteria that could be educating her immune system. In a home like the one where Jack raised his kids, the mold and fungus could have been damaging. But by opening the windows and doors most of the time, and by spending a lot of time outside, it's possible that negative side effects of living in a confined indoor environment could have been ameliorated. And the input of good bacteria and maybe even good fungi from outside may have helped reduce the opportunity for the bad ones to grow.

Given evidence that soil and animal microbes can help build a healthy immune system, at least in mice, exposing your child to fresh air is probably a good plan.

13

Conditions

My child has a weird rash. Is the microbiome involved?

Oddly we get variants of this question all the time. And as you might expect, they are very hard to answer. Any time your child's immune system is out of balance, he may be susceptible to other conditions, including skin infections.

The term "generic rash" is used to describe many different diseases. The problem is that most skin diseases are difficult to diagnose as the manifestation is always the same—a weird rash.

Your child's skin, like his gut, has a diverse and complex microbiome. In fact, the microbiome varies all over his skin, with chemical and biological differences driven by the amount of oil or moisture that is found there. So the dry parts of human skin have a very different microbiome than the moist areas. Rob's lab has worked with collaborators to figure out the differences in adults, but young children have not yet been examined for this.

Skin diseases are another matter. Changes in your skin microbiome (or your child's) may be diagnostic for a variety of skin disorders. But dermatologists have a long way to go in working this out. And sometimes very simple solutions present themselves.

For example, Jack developed a weird rash while he lived and worked in the Antarctic between 1999 and 2001. Around twelve months into the expedition, the rash appeared and eventually spread all over his body. The medical professional on base opined that it was a fungal infection. He gave Jack some antifungal medicine. Jack asked how he knew, and he replied "I don't, but everyone gets those down here, so it might be!" A very unsatisfactory answer.

When the boat came down to take him home, it also brought a group of new researchers and maintenance staff, including a new doctor. She just so happened to be a dermatologist. As soon as she was set up, Jack went and asked her what she thought the rash could be. Her response was only slightly better than that given by the first doc. "Well, it looks viral, but there is no way to be sure; I suggest you use some moisturizer daily and it will probably take care of itself."

There was no test that could explain the condition, no diagnosis, and basically no treatment. Instead, Jack was to hydrate his skin and wait for things to get better. Remarkably, they did. To this day Jack assumes that moisturizing his skin helped to reset the playing field and enabled his immune system to take care of the infection. If the doctors had been able to determine how the microbiome had altered on his skin, they might have been able to fix the problem much sooner or even come up with a more specific therapy. As it happened, that was not necessary.

But for other conditions it could be. Skin wounds are constantly at risk of infection. Bacteria can invade exposed tissues, offering a ripe environment for breeding and nasty infections. Some of these bacteria, such as *Staphylococcus*, live on the skin and take advantage of the new situation. Others can be introduced from outside, such as necrotizing fasciitis, or flesh-eating bacteria. While the latter is rare, the results are extreme. From our perspective, what's more interesting is that your skin's microbiome can play a role in defending you and your child against these pathogens. The microbiome in general may play a role in helping the body to heal a wound.

For the most part bacteria in a wound appear to slow down healing. We know this because wounds tend to heal faster on a germ-free animal than they do in a mouse full of bacteria. But even more intriguingly, mice with a skin wound that are fed a live probiotic appear to heal faster than those fed dead bacteria. This suggests that our old friend the immune system may be responding to the gut bacterial infusion and somehow stimulating wound healing. The mechanism is unknown, but the results are fascinating and beg further analysis.

If there are disease-causing bacteria in my child's throat (nose, etc.), why don't they make him sick?

This may surprise to you, but healthy people routinely carry around microbes that can act as pathogens—with no ill effect.[1] We have a deep fear of germs known to cause disease, but in most cases they are friendly passengers on the human bus.

This was seen in the nineteenth century with tuberculosis, a particularly dreaded disease that killed millions of people each year. Robert Koch, a celebrated German physician and pioneering microbiologist, developed a set of postulates for proving microbes cause disease. First, prove the microbe is found in sick people. Then show it isn't found in healthy people. Next, show that you can isolate the organism and infect healthy people with it so that they fall sick. The procedure didn't work for tuberculosis, the main microbe he studied, because many apparently healthy people carry the microbe.

Mary Mallong (known as Typhoid Mary) is another notorious

case. Mary worked as a cook in the New York City region for seven affluent families. Although she had no symptoms of typhoid fever, she shed the bacteria into her employers' food every day, sickening and killing many (but, interestingly, not all) of them. Mary refused to believe she was the cause of so much mayhem and had to be quarantined multiple times.

Changes in diet, microbiome, or immune status can affect whether any pathogen—be it a bacterium, virus, or parasite—will colonize an animal or cause harm if it does colonize. The same is probably true for people, though this remains to be studied in detail.

Competition between microbes may also shed light on why pathogens do or don't make us sick. You've probably heard of staph infections—caused by *Staphylococcus aureus*. It can lurk in your child's nose as a harmless bug. But when some kids get sick, or go into the hospital for surgery, or if their immune system becomes suppressed, then this harmless bug can perform a Jekyll-and-Hyde transformation to become harmful. *S. aureus* can activate pathogenic genes in its genome that take advantage of a child's lowered defenses. These staph infections can often be eliminated by antibiotics; but over the last twenty years we have seen an increase in the number of people harboring a strain of *S. aureus* that is resistant to the antibiotics we use to kill them, such as methicillin. We call this new strain methicillin-resistant *Staphylococcus aureus*, or MRSA. When your child's defenses are down, this bug can lead to life-threatening infections that do not respond to standard antibiotics.

However, some children who harbor either strain, normal or resistant staph, do not get infected. Somehow they are protected.

In a recent study, scientists found that children who have another species of *Staphylococcus*, *S. lugdunensis*, in their noses seem to have some protection from staph infections.[2]

S. lugdunensis produces a microbial antibiotic that kills off the *S. aureus*. It's a matter of simple competition. *S. lugdunensis* has found a way of clearing out competitors so that it can predominate. This is not all good news as *S. lugdunensis* can itself cause skin infections. But these are much less common than *S. aureus*.

Either way—just because your child carries a pathogen doesn't mean he will come down with a disease. Most diseases result from a perfect storm: your child is infected and susceptible, and all the right (or wrong) conditions come together and he gets sick. Unfortunately, this outcome is really hard to predict, and we still don't know much about it.

I read somewhere that microbes can cause obesity. Is that true?

Yes, at least in mice. Mice can get fat for a lot of different reasons, mostly caused by scientists. They can have genetic defects that make them tubby. Or they can be fed a bad diet. Amazingly, in both these cases, the microbiome changes in ways that lead to increased inflammation, glucose intolerance, and ultimately even diabetes. And what's even more amazing is that you can take that microbiome and transplant it into another mouse that's raised germ-free, with no microbes of its own. That mouse will then become fat even if it doesn't have the genetic defect or the bad diet. This shows that microbes can transmit obesity.

The same transmission hasn't been shown in humans—yet. As of now, we have lots of evidence hinting that it might be possible. For example, if you have many overweight friends, you're likely to be fatter yourself. If you're heavier, your dog is likely to be chubby too, and we know that humans and dogs exchange microbes with each other all the time. Moreover, obese people, including children, have different microbiomes than lean people.

A lot of this work has been carried out by Rob's collaborator, Jeffrey I. Gordon, at Washington University, and his former trainees, including Ruth Ley, now at the Max Planck Institute. We used to think, based on mouse studies and one early human study, that the ratio of two types of bacteria, the Firmicutes and the Bacteroidetes, was the most important explanation for obesity. More Firmicutes compared to Bacteroidetes was considered to be predictive of obesity.

Recent work has shown that the condition is more likely to be related to an energy imbalance, rather than just the imbalance of these two types of bacteria. You can tell whether someone's lean or obese with up to 90 percent accuracy simply by looking at his or her microbiome, at least within the context of a single study.

Does this mean that a microbiome-based test for obesity is coming soon? Well, probably not. It's a lot easier to weigh yourself and measure your height than it is to sequence your microbiome. Also, differences between the ways in which studies measure the microbiome and in how people are defined as lean or obese (including whether prediabetes or other metabolic problems are observed) can lead to subtle differences between populations that make a universal test hard to achieve right now.

Even more amazing is that you can transfer human microbes into mice to make them fatter. That's right: mice that get microbes from an overweight person become heavier. This even works if instead of transferring the poop, you grow hundreds of strains of bacteria from a single person's feces, then transfer that into a mouse. This proves that the bacteria are doing the job— not viruses, not chemicals transferred along with the poop, not antibodies or anything else.

So does this mean the microbiome can make your child fat? Much less work has been done on obese children than obese adults in terms of the microbiome, although several studies have reported differences. One interesting observation comes from Dr. Martin Blaser's lab at NYU. Researchers found that the combination of C-section and antibiotics in early life increases the risk of obesity later on. This effect can be partly counteracted by breast-feeding and a diet consisting of a diverse array of brightly colored plants. These are two things that are under parental control and can be implemented now, without waiting for any additional research. We know that microbes are involved in all of these processes. So stay tuned for microbiome discoveries related to childhood obesity.

> I heard that my son's asthma was caused by a lack of microbial exposure. Is this true? What can I do about it?

Asthma is a chronic lung condition, although the same symptoms (labored breathing due to constricting muscles around inflamed airways) can sometimes be induced in nonasthmatics if they exercise too hard. Asthma is one of those conditions that is often discussed under the general category of atopy, which is basically an inappropriate inflammation gone rogue. This inflammation can be triggered by an otherwise innocuous allergen, just like food, seasonal changes, and skin allergies.

We know that people who grow up in households with less microbial diversity have an increased risk of developing asthma, although exposure to microbes is only one of many factors that contributes to this complex disease. For reasons we don't fully understand, children who grow up with dogs have a 13 percent reduction in the likelihood of developing asthma.[3] Dogs also sport a lot of their own bacteria; in one animal study that exposed mice to dog-associated house dust, the mice were protected from asthma attacks. Mice exposed to this dog dust also show a significantly altered gut microbiome, with more of a microbe called *L. johnsonii*. This bacterium, when given to the mice as an edible probiotic, also protects them from having an asthma-like reaction.[4]

In another study, Jack and his collaborators took house dust from the homes of Amish and Hutterite families and exposed mice to both samples.[5] Dust from the Amish home protected mice against an asthma-like reaction, whereas the Hutterite dust was not protective. Something in the Amish dust appears protective. While the results are not definitive, the microbial communities found in each of these dust samples was different. We have reason to believe that the constant exposure Amish households get from living on farms with many animals likely produces a different microbial community, especially when compared to the Hutterites who do not live on farms, despite both groups living a mostly technology-free existence.

However, if your child has asthma, don't blame yourself for providing an inadequate environment. Short of moving to a farm and living an Amish lifestyle (or, better yet, becoming a hunter-gatherer), it's very hard to predict if a child will get asthma. And there might be other drawbacks to such radically different life-styles, such as your kid being kicked by a horse or eaten by hyenas.

In another study, researchers found that infants who developed asthma had a period of microbiome disruption within their first hundred days of life. In comparing their microbiomes to kids who did not develop asthma, they found that four types of bacteria—*Lachnospira*, *Veillonella*, *Faecalibacterium*, and *Rothia*—were nearly absent in the asthmatic kids. When they grew these bacteria in the lab and gave them to mice, the animals were protected against asthma's airway inflammation.[6]

As with the *Lactobacillus* that was induced by the dog dust, there is something about these four bacteria that helps to protect a person's airways from becoming inflamed. The current hypothesis is that they help regulate inflammation. They do this by producing certain chemicals (short-chain fatty acids) that feed the immune system and help it to keep a lid on inflammation.

In a recent study, researchers found that by-products of gut microbes in some month-old infants trigger inflammation that is linked to their becoming allergy prone by age two and asthmatic by age four.[7] The babies have abnormally low levels of four kinds of commensal or friendly microbes (*Bifidobacteria, Lactobacillus, Faecalibacterium, and Akkermansia*) and higher relative levels of two types of fungi. Together their metabolites skew immune function.

Once asthma has developed, it's difficult to treat. However, there has never been any real understanding of why. Again, the microbiome comes in. It seems as if some of these bacteria that work on baby mice don't protect adult mice from airway inflammation. One reason could be that the animals' existing microbiomes are too robust, and the probiotics just can't find a home in the gut to do their job. In children or young animals, the microbiome is quite dynamic and tends to be less diverse, so it is easier for new organisms introduced in a probiotic to get a foothold.

Finally, diet may help control symptoms by interacting with microbes and the immune system. Some studies find that correcting vitamin D deficiencies and encouraging a healthy diet, such as the Mediterranean diet, can be beneficial.

How does the microbiome affect my child's autism?

As the father of an autistic son, Jack has a unique perspective on this. His son, Dylan, is higher functioning and although he struggles with concepts and has some difficulty with contexts, he is still a happy kid with friends. He loves being with people, and sometimes he doesn't. In many ways he is very normal, but he sometimes struggles to fit into the version of society that we have created.

Autism spectrum disorder is a developmental condition affecting one in sixty-eight children in the United States. Kids and adults show a broad range of behavioral and physiological symptoms. For reasons we cannot yet explain, the prevalence of autism seems to be rising. Fifty years ago, it was one in ten thousand. We know it is highly heritable, passing down through generations of families. While there are many candidate genes that could play a role in some of the neurological and physiological attributes of the condition, there is also plenty of evidence pointing to environmental triggers.

Before we go further, we want to say something about the term "disorder." Many autistic children on the spectrum are more "normal" than you might think. They do well in school and grow up to fall in love, have families, hold down a job, and be highly productive members of society. At the lower, more severe end of the spectrum, kids may bang their heads against the wall, rock incessantly, flap their arms as if to confirm their existence, lack speech, be unable to make eye contact, and erupt in violent temper tantrums. Many have severe gastrointestinal issues, including diarrhea, colitis, and leaky gut—a breakdown in their gut wall integrity that allows bacteria and their chemicals to leak out.

When scientists carry out human experiments, it's incredibly difficult to deal with a spectrum disorder. Think about it. People are incredibly diverse and have a remarkable range of lifestyles and personal histories. All could influence the variation in symptoms. So when trying to uncover factors that influence variability—between, say, patients with autism spectrum disorder and those without—the fact that autism is itself so variable makes the analysis next to impossible. Treating autism as a discrete disorder rather than as a collection of many different forms means that attempts to search for genes, lifestyle factors, or indeed the microbiome are very difficult and probably not important. Moreover, the genes linked to autism account for only about 40 percent of the variability in symptoms. This suggests that as much as 60 percent of the difference in symptoms across the spectrum may be related to environmental factors, including the microbiome.

Recently, a possible treatment for autism spectrum disorder involving gut microbe, probiotics, and a mouse model of the condition made the news. The animals have stereotypical behaviors and physiological symptoms similar to those seen in autistic children, including a leaky gut and elevated levels of certain metabolites (chemicals) produced by bacteria in blood and urine.[8] When researchers gave the probiotic *Bacteroides fragilis* to the mice, some of their key behavioral and physical symptoms were alleviated.

That a probiotic can do this for a mouse doesn't necessarily mean that it can work in children—but it might. These results have led researchers to wonder if children across the spectrum are maybe missing certain bacteria that could be added back into their bodies as a probiotic. Early investigations suggest that children diagnosed with autism have an increased abundance of the bacterial genus *Clostridium*, and a reduction in the abundance of *Bifidobacterium* and *Prevotella*; therefore, maybe we could develop a new therapy by augmenting the children's microbiome with *Bifidobacterium* and *Prevotella*.[9] This corroborates what the mouse model showed—that adding back bacteria such as *Bifidobacterium* and *Prevotella* could be beneficial in reducing the symptoms of autism.

We're a long way from finding a solution, but using prebiotics to change the abundance of beneficial gut bacteria such as *Bifidobacterium* and *Prevotella* is a start. These are predominant fermenters that can be supported by eating more fibers that provide the carbohydrates that will feed these bacteria. Alternatively, consuming *Bifidobacterium* as a probiotic may help—although there is no clinical evidence to support this claim right now. *Bifidobacterium* has been used as a probiotic for more than a hundred years and has shown no adverse side effects. Probiotics may be easier than diet modifications as the parent of any child with autism will tell you; like most, they're picky eaters. But in the early stages of life—under age three—it may be possible to augment their diet and improve symptoms.

Clearly we need a better understanding of diet-microbiome relationships in association with brain-behavioral disturbances. Some children are sensitive to gluten, dairy/casein, and histamine-rich foods or other food allergens. You should work with a reputable allergist and nutritionist to address such problems. Kids with GI inflammatory issues can benefit from a low carbohydrate diet or the ketogenic diet (the latter especially for kids with seizure disorder comorbidities). It is difficult to generalize from the individual experiences posted by parents online to what you should do for children in general, because every case is so different. However, as we get a better understanding of the underlying conditions, their links to the microbiome, and the role of diet, it is likely that more useful advice will emerge.

Jack has never tried to impose a regimented diet on Dylan. He's just not that type of child. However, Jack and his wife have found ways to ensure a healthy diet, composed of fresh vegetables and fruit and avoidance of refined sugar. That being said, Dylan still gets to eat his favorite cereal and sometimes has too much candy. He is a kid after all. But there is fallout from these splurges, often culminating in behavioral outbursts that can be upsetting for everyone.

Jack has seen a few circumstantial reports on fecal microbiome transplants to treat autism spectrum disorder. But these procedures have been performed on older children, and the limited scope of the investigations leaves the interpretation of results in question. Don't do it yourself at home until much more information is available, as the risks are considerable and the benefits are at this point unclear.

Can the oral microbiome tell me if my child is at risk for cavities?

Yes. Early childhood cavities are the most common infection in children. A study carried out in China that Rob's lab collaborated on tracked microbes in plaque and saliva in fifty four-year-old preschoolers for two years.[10] Children either stayed healthy, started developing cavities, or got cavities. They saw clear differences in the types and abundance of oral microbes in each group and could even predict the appearance of cavities several months in advance—with over 80 percent accuracy.

Testing whether the prediction works in other populations, including the United States, is still a work in progress. But one day you might be able to test whether your kid is at risk for cavities by getting him to spit in a cup and then sequencing his bacteria.

How can I tell if my child is developing celiac disease or gluten intolerance? Is the microbiome involved?

Celiac disease is a genetically based autoimmune condition in which gluten, a specific protein in wheat and several other grains, causes the immune system to shred the cells lining the gut. If tissue transglutaminase antibodies are present in your child's blood, then it is extremely likely that he has the disease. The test is 98 percent accurate if his diet includes gluten. (It doesn't work if he's on a gluten-free diet.) A clinical diagnosis requires a tissue biopsy—a rather invasive and drastic procedure. The physician inserts an endoscope into your child's intestine and clips off a small piece of tissue to examine under a microscope. So, if he has been diagnosed with celiac disease he has been through the wringer already.

The gastrointestinal lining of patients with celiac disease has a distinct microbiome, showing a relatively greater abundance of Proteobacteria.[11] This is probably in response to inflammation stemming from the immune system mounting a defense against gluten. Celiac patients whose disease symptoms do not respond to a gluten-free diet may have this sort of abnormal microbiome, but animal studies to confirm the hypothesis have not been done. There's reason to hope that antibiotic therapy combined with probiotic or fecal microbiome transplant might be able to reset the celiac microbiome.

It's still hotly debated whether so-called gluten intolerance, as opposed to celiac disease, really exists. The assertion is that some people are sensitive to gluten, suggesting a mild allergic reaction and inflammatory response to foods containing gluten. This is hard to prove because the symptoms are vague and attempts to look for inflamed tissue via a colonoscopy don't seem to support some of the claims.

We can find no evidence that gluten intolerance is related to changes in your child's microbiome. People who eliminate gluten from their diet change their carbohydrate intake and other parameters that affect health and mood, so it is difficult to isolate the effects of gluten per se.

My child has diabetes. Is the microbiome involved?

Yes. And it's another reason why dirt is good for your baby. Juvenile or type 1 diabetes is a chronic condition in which your child's pancreas produces little or no insulin—a hormone that allows sugar, or glucose, to enter the body's cells and produce energy. Symptoms include increased thirst, frequent urination, bedwetting in kids who previously did not wet the bed, extreme hunger, weight loss, mood changes, and fatigue. Some of these symptoms can show up in babies or kids under three, but you should also look for disorientation and blurred vision, and their breath can smell like wine. The exact cause of the disease is not known. In any case, your child's immune system turns against itself and destroys insulin-producing cells in the pancreas. Sugar builds up in your child's bloodstream, creating life-threatening complications.

Several genes linked to the immune system make type 1 diabetes more likely to occur. However, these genes can't explain why type 1 diabetes is increasing so rapidly around the world, because there hasn't been enough time for these genes to change in frequency. Risk factors include low vitamin D (which is involved in immune system function), the age at which gluten is introduced into the diet (before four months or after seven months seem to be problematic), and some viral infections. An ongoing study of thousands of high-risk children is currently looking for more risk factors, including the microbiome.

Type 2 diabetes is also a chronic metabolic disorder caused by resistance to insulin. The incidence of this disease has been sky-rocketing in children, coinciding with the sharp rise in childhood obesity. Nowadays type 2 diabetes accounts for up to one-third of childhood cases and is particularly common in at-risk populations: minority, overweight, and pubescent children.

In type 2 diabetes, resistance to insulin develops, so even though it is being produced, the body doesn't respond to it. Although insulin injections can be used as a last resort, they can further accelerate the process of insulin resistance. Instead, diet (high-fiber, low-sugar, rich in fruits and vegetables) and exercise are the first line of treatment. A drug called metformin is being used in children to improve their body's sensitivity to insulin. Since metformin itself affects the microbiome, we can't tell what is cause and what is effect. In extreme cases of obesity, bariatric surgery—in which the stomach is reduced in size and the digestive tract rearranged—is often recommended for adults. It has a dramatic effect on insulin sensitivity, restoring function in just a couple of days far in advance of any weight loss. Interestingly, all of these factors have strong effects on the microbiome.

We know a lot more about the relationship between type 2 diabetes and the microbiome. In mice, microbiome changes induced by genetic changes, diet, artificial sweeteners, and even disrupted sleep can lead to insulin resistance. The trait can be transplanted via poop from one mouse to another, or even from diabetic humans into mice. In these experiments, germ-free mice are the stool recipients. Researchers are trying to figure out which are the most important individual bacteria or combinations of bacteria involved in transferring insulin resistance. Encouragingly, one study in the Netherlands showed that transplanting stool from lean to obese donors helped to restore insulin sensitivity, although it did little for the obesity. Does this mean you should get a stool transplant for your child's diabetes? No, but it does suggest that therapies based on the microbiome may be in the future.

· · · · · · · · ·

The current mystery is why the prevalence of type 1 and type 2 diabetes is rising so rapidly around the world. In the United States, the CDC reports that diabetes prevalence has more than doubled since 1980. As noted, there has not been enough time for genes to change their frequency in the human population. Therefore, a nongenetic component must be involved.

Several years ago, a team of scientists started following thirty-three newborns who were genetically at risk of developing type 1 diabetes.[12] They were born in Finland, which has the highest prevalence of type 1 diabetes in the world. Nearly 1 in 120 kids under the age of fifteen has it. By age three, four of the kids in the study were diabetic. In looking at how the children developed, the scientists discovered a set of common changes a year before the disease appeared, including autoantibodies—immune cells that attack the body's own tissues. The diversity of gut microbes declined as a set of inflammatory microbes bloomed.

The researchers wondered if they could slow down or correct this process, so they conducted a follow-up study. They identified 222 newborns who were genetically at risk for developing type 1 diabetes from three countries—Finland, Estonia, and Russia. The Russians were from Karelia, the region across the Finnish border, with both sides having similar environments. By age three, sixteen Finnish and fourteen Estonian kids had autoantibodies and excess sugar in their blood. Only four Russian children did.

Then they looked at their microbial profiles, and clear differences stood out. The guts of both Finnish and Estonian children were dominated by *Bacteroides*. The Russian kids showed high levels of *Bifidobacteria* and *E. coli*.

Drilling down, the scientists looked at how those microbes functioned. Some bacteria, including the ones found in the kids, make a by-product called endotoxin—a toxin found inside a bacterial cell that is released when the cell disintegrates. Endotoxin prompts white blood cells into action. Endotoxins from the Russian microbes would do Putin proud. They strongly stimulated the children's immune cells in a way that induced self-tolerance—that is, the immune cells would not attack the body's own proteins and other antigens. But the Finnish and Estonian endotoxin was comparatively inert. In a set of mouse experiments, white blood cells didn't notice the endotoxin. (It failed to protect the mice from developing diabetes.)

Why was Russian microbiome different? It wasn't food. The kids ate similar diets, though the Russians had less packaged goods. Breast-feeding was similar. But one difference did stand out. The Russians were poorer. Their well water was untreated. Their homes were shabbier. They lacked the accoutrements of advanced Western countries like dishwashers and Dyson vacuum cleaners. The upshot: Russian homes contained a more diverse community of microbes.

This finding is another example of the hygiene hypothesis. It is also another example of why we need to understand how a more complex microbial exposure early in life can protect people from developing these conditions. Unless we all want to go back to living in less pleasant settings, we had better figure out how to improve that microbial exposure in a more artificial way.

> How can I best deal with constant ear infections? How can I break the cycle?

Antibiotics do very little for ear infections. They may reduce symptoms for a day or two at best. At the same time, they are likely to disrupt your child's microbiome and set them up for more health problems later, including additional ear infections.

You can take other steps to minimize the risk of ear infections by eliminating exposure to cigarette smoke and by asking day-care staff to recommend that sick kids stay home. You can also maximize protective factors such as breast-feeding (if feasible and appropriate) and use probiotics.

Ear infections are commonly caused by bacteria and viruses that promote inflammation in the inner ear. As with many other conditions we have discussed, inflammation can be controlled by adding bacteria back into the gut. While we don't necessarily understand why certain probiotics do this, they do appear to work. Importantly, this can be achieved with probiotics from the pharmacy, even if the organisms in these probiotics do not necessarily have the functional capacity themselves to reduce inflammation. Some of these off-the-shelf probiotics (such as *Lactobacillus rhamnosus* GG) seem to stimulate the growth of bacteria in the gut that can help to suppress inflammation.

So giving your child a probiotic when he has an earache may help to relieve some of the symptoms.

> Can doctors run tests in their offices to determine if an infection is bacterial or viral?

Sorry, not yet. Tests to determine if an infection is bacterial or viral are too slow to run in the doctor's office. The gold standard for identifying a bacterium is culturing—placing a sample such as fluid from a throat swab onto a nutrient and waiting to see if bacteria grow out. This typically takes three days to a week, longer than you'd want to hang around a doctor's office. Tests based on DNA sequencing are faster but still take a day or two. A technique called quantitative PCR (qPCR), which is DNA-based and looks at specific markers, can theoretically be done in a few hours, but fast versions are not currently FDA-approved. Some new tests that look at how blood cells activate their genes can be used to distinguish bacterial and viral infections, but these assays are not approved by the FDA.

When Rob's daughter got a skin rash from staph, he was frustrated about the gap between what was possible in a research lab versus what was standard clinical practice. They took her in to get the infection looked at right before the New Year's holiday and were told it would take three days to get the result, but meanwhile here were some antibiotics. First thing in the morning of January 2, they got a panicked phone call from the clinic: the rash was caused by antibiotic-resistant staph, the antibiotics wouldn't work, and they needed to come in for a new prescription. That was fascinating, because the antibiotics had in fact worked. So it had taken the standard microbiological testing three days to come up with the wrong answer. In contrast, the kinds of PCR-based assays now done in the field can be performed in a few hours using a handheld unit, and complete genome sequencing can be done faster than the culture-based assays now. Rob is now working hard to figure out how to bring these advances into the clinic so that other families don't have to go through what his family did. But validation and regulatory approval is a painstaking and slow process.

So there is hope that such a test may one day be possible, but it isn't right now.

What is a fecal matter transfer and might it help treat my child's medical issue?

A fecal matter transplant, or fecal microbiome transplant (FMT) is exactly what it sounds like. We know that organ transplants can cure many diseases. An FMT aims to replace a broken gut microbiome with one that functions properly. In this sense, your gut microbiome may be viewed like a heart, liver, or kidney. Although the analogy is not perfect, it helps explain how an FMT works.

In the procedure, stool taken from a healthy person is mixed with sterile water and then inserted into the colon of a person whose gut is in trouble. It can be delivered via a nasal tube into the upper colon, via an enema, or in capsule form. Whether it works depends on the recipient having a genuine disorder of the microbiome and empty ecological niches to fill. It might also depend on the microbiome of the donor, although the evidence is less clear on this right now.

One particular problem—an infection caused by the gut bacterium *Clostridium difficile*—responds amazingly well to an FMT. In one well-controlled study, patients who got the treatment experienced a 94 percent cure rate compared to a success rate of 35 percent in those who received the standard treatment: a dose of vancomycin, an antibiotic that is not absorbed into the gut wall and is designed to perform a blitzkrieg on the gut bacteria. When the blitzkrieg failed and the FMT worked spectacularly well, the patients who took the antibiotic got the fecal transfer right away. It was deemed unethical to continue treating them with the drug.

So how does the FMT work? While the organ-transplant analogy is appealing, it's slightly misleading. A better analogy might be one that is technically speaking impossible. Let's say we wanted to rebuild a rain forest: how would we do it? One way might be to get seeds from all the plants and eggs or parents for all the animals, and then put them in some bare soil and see what happens. Trust us: this won't work. A rain forest is a very complex ecosystem, with a huge number of interconnections, and it takes a long time to establish them. While the forest is developing it goes through many different phases, and no two rain forests are alike. Sounds rather like the human microbiome right? Well, the only way to replace a rain forest in one go would be to pick up another rain forest from a similar place and put it into the space where the old one used to be. Basically, you are replacing an absent or dysfunctional ecosystem with a fully functional, complex ecosystem.

The problem is, we don't exactly understand how or why a complex ecosystem works. Faced with so many moving parts, we've not been able to tease apart what each bit does and how the many interactions culminate to produce the effects we see. So instead of building a fully functioning microbiome from scratch, it is much easier to just replace it with an existing one.

FMT has been tried on a number of other diseases. For example, an ongoing clinical trial at the University of Pittsburgh is looking to see if FMT can help children with inflammatory bowel diseases, Crohn's disease, and ulcerative colitis. Another study from the University of Florida is examining the role of microbial disturbance in obese infants and mothers where FMT may someday help. You can find out about these studies by going to www.clinicaltrials.gov and searching "microbiome, pediatric." Forty-two current or planned trials fit this description.

At the time of this writing, the FDA only approves FMT to

help with recurrent *C. difficile* infections. To treat other conditions, clinicians must obtain an investigative new drug license, which can be cumbersome and expensive. The situation may change in the next few years.

14

....

Tests

Are there risks to having my child's stool tested?

There aren't any risks to having your child's stool tested (at least to you). You're handling your child's poop all the time anyway, and you won't have to touch it to get it tested because you collect samples with a cotton swab or by having them poop into a container.

Theoretically there could be privacy concerns, but babies' microbiomes change so fast that a sample collected later on can't be traced back to them even if the data were released. A lot of this relies on the type of data you generate, of course. The 16S rRNA data (discussed later) are not refined enough to be able to make predictions at this time. The metagenomic data could potentially be used to trace a sample back to an individual. That being said, these data are very well protected, with privacy governed by strict federal laws. It would be an extraordinary situation if someone were able to acquire a sample, trace it to an individual, and then somehow use that information against the person. In fact, neither of us could conceive of what they would do with that data anyway.

One potential issue, as with any medical testing, is that an inconclusive or incorrect result could prompt you to take action that might be unnecessary, such as an extreme diet or medical intervention. For that reason, anything you find out using the microbiome should be complemented with FDA-approved medical tests.

Should I get my microbiome tested before I get pregnant?

If you're worried about infertility, the links between your microbiome (especially your vaginal and urinary microbiome) and an inability to conceive are weak, so there's no compelling reason to get yours tested before trying to get pregnant. However, having your oral microbiome explored before conceiving may be a good idea. We know that preterm birth is linked to poor oral hygiene; it's likely triggered by bacteria entering your bloodstream from bleeding gums and causing inflammation when they reach the placenta. Instead of having your microbiome sequenced, you may want to see a dentist to ensure that you have no gum disease or tooth decay.

That said, it may one day be possible to track changes in your microbiome before you get pregnant to predict problems before they happen. This is an exciting direction of research. For example, we hope to be able to use the vaginal microbiome during early pregnancy or even before pregnancy to predict whether a mother is likely to give birth preterm, develop gestational diabetes, or suffer from perinatal depression. We are not there yet, because we need to feed a lot more data into our algorithms before we can give credence to our predictions.

The future is bright though. We know there are many other risk factors that are already being used to make similar predictions. The more things you can measure, the easier it will be to predict differences between people and outcomes. Hence, adding microbiome to the list of other factors (history of preterm birth, dental hygiene, weight, BMI, etc.) will help us to refine predictions and improve our ability to offer precision health care.

> If I decide to get my child's microbiome tested, how do I go about doing it?

An increasing number of options for testing your child's microbiome are popping up. Research projects such as the American Gut Project, which we run, allow you to use the same techniques employed by many large-scale research projects, including the Earth Microbiome Project—a collaborative effort to sequence and characterize the microbiome of planet Earth (cofounded by us as well). But the laboratory and computational protocols in these large-scale projects have been used and cited in literally thousands of scientific studies. If you want to explore American Gut as an option, more information can be found at www.americangut.org.

To collect a sample, you dip a cotton swab into some of your child's poop—usually from a diaper, but let's face it, the poop doesn't always go into the diaper so you can swab it from anywhere—and mail it in. You'll get back a readout of the kinds of bacteria and other microbes from your child's gut, based on a technique called 16S rRNA gene sequencing used to identify bacterial species. (More elaborate forms of sequencing that look at the viruses, the rest of the genome, and even the rest of the RNA can also be done through American Gut.) We also compare your microbiome to the more than ten thousand other samples that we have already processed. This allows you to see how your child's microbiome compares to other children their age or with similar diets. It's also possible to compare your child's microbiome to other children with similar conditions.

All software and data from the project are open-source, so they can be shared by other researchers and used to find out more about your microbiome. More importantly, because all the methods are published and subject to scrutiny by the whole scientific community, the results are generally robust and reliable. By taking part in the American Gut Project, you are supporting researchers around the world by providing a reliable data set that they can access and use to explore how the microbiome varies between individuals.

Think about it this way. We have explained many times how some of the studies we report on in this book are often based on only a small number of patients. So a study that finds a bacterial species that appears to be more abundant in children with Crohn's disease may seem exciting. If that study only compares twenty children with Crohn's and twenty without, however, the ability to extrapolate these findings to your individual child is limited. But if those researchers can then explore the American Gut database and find that this bacterium is abundant in all the children identified with Crohn's, this lends meaningful support to their findings. They can then use this combined evidence to apply for funding to support a larger study or to advance their investigation to a clinical trial.

Companies such as uBiome, Whole Biome, Second Genome, and many others use the same general principles, but they have modified the protocols in proprietary ways. This means that you can't easily compare their results to published studies. And because their software is not open-source, it has not been verified by the wider scientific community. Hence their results are less certain. Also, your results, while not shared with other researchers, are used by the company to make money, usually by selling them to pharmaceutical companies.

If you decide to get your child's microbiome sequenced, you might want to know a bit more about the strategies we use. As mentioned above, 16S rRNA gene sequencing is used to distinguish bacterial species. It is simply the DNA of a single gene that is found in all bacteria. We use it like a barcode: with it we can tell how many species there are in a sample and roughly identify the names of those species.

In the metagenomic method we sequence all the genes in all of the microbes in a sample. It's akin to the Human Genome Project where we've been able to explore your genetic blueprint—all the DNA that codes for all the proteins and structures in your body. Similarly, metagenomic sequencing allows us to read the blueprint for all the bacteria in your gut. Whereas 16S rRNA amplicon sequencing tells us roughly who is there, metagenomic sequencing tells us what those microbes are capable of doing. This is a better way of investigating your child's microbiome.

By looking at all the genes, from all the microbes in a sample, we can start to reconstruct how the bacteria in your child's gut may respond to a certain diet, or why your child's microbiome may be causing excess inflammation in her intestine. The genomes of each microbe contain information that we can use to predict what foods the bacteria like to eat and what chemicals they are likely to excrete.

Jack has a story that sheds light on how such tests can be used: Around 2014, he was suffering from joint pain in his fingers. His doctor diagnosed a mild form of arthritis and recommended he take a steroid. He was not overly convinced by this. Steroids are supposed to bring down inflammation in blood vessels and muscle, and many people with chronic arthritis use the drug to improve their quality of life. But he was thirty-seven years old and not quite ready to accept that fate.

He had recently lost a lot of weight, reducing his mass from 205 pounds to 165 pounds in around twelve weeks using a strict regimen of diet and exercise. He had examined his microbes before and after and noted that, naturally, things had changed. He had been eating different foods and exercising more, so his whole body had shifted along with his microbiome. But he wondered if something in his microbiome might give a clue as to what caused the inflammation in his fingers. When he sequenced his microbiome over seven days he noticed that he had an excess abundance of *Bacteroides*. This is a common gut microbe that tends to feed on sugar, but it was rather too abundant. We often see it blooming when you have diarrhea or a leaky gut, as the gut's ability to absorb sugar starts to fail. More sugar in the gut means more *Bacteroides* can grow. He could see this pattern using metagenomics: the genomes of the *Bacteroides* in his gut contained all the genes needed to consume many different types of sugar. It's possible, although not provable, that all the exercise he had been doing was causing inflammation in his body—he had been pushing it rather hard—and that this inflammation may have led to malabsorption of sugar in his gut, leading to the overgrowth of *Bacteroides*.

But he had a more likely explanation, albeit one he was not willing to admit to. He had lost a lot of weight and was exercising more, but he didn't want to lose any more weight. As he was counting his calories, he knew exactly how much energy he was burning and how much he was consuming. His aim was to ensure that his weight stayed around 165 to170 pounds, so he was trying to balance the number of calories he consumed with the number he burned. But he found it hard to balance exercise and work and getting all the calories he needed to stay on course. So he turned to candy bars. He bought large quantities of his favorite Cadbury chocolate candy bars and ate a lot of them each day to make up his calories. Although he has no proof of this, there was a very interesting correlation between the increase in sugar-loving bugs in his gut and his practice of eating sugar to get enough calories. And this, of course, coincided with his systemic inflammation and joint pain. Sugar has been linked to inflammation in many other studies, and low-sugar diets are recommended for a range of autoimmune and inflammatory conditions.

So Jack stopped eating the chocolate bars and started eating more protein snacks and vegetables to make up for the calorie shortage. Right away he saw a reduction in the abundance of *Bacteroides* in his gut and, within three weeks, his joint pain went away. This is a complex story, but we tell it to show you how understanding the microbes in your gut can be helpful in figuring out a way to change your diet and maybe influence your health.

We want to make it clear that this is not an easy process. Jack has extraordinary resources and expertise at his fingertips, so he can explore ways to manipulate his diet. Also, these testing techniques cost a lot of money. While 16S rRNA amplicon sequencing is relatively cheap (around $75 a sample), metagenomics, when done properly, usually costs a lot more (around $500 a sample) and takes more time to analyze. Sometimes this can take many hundreds of hours on a supercomputer; this doesn't translate to hundreds of hours in real life as the supercomputer runs everything at the same time on different processors. But still, it's expensive.

The hope is that these metagenomic studies will help us improve our ability to interpret the cheaper 16S rRNA amplicon studies. We can compare what each technique shows and advance our ability to make useful and practicable interpretations from these data.

Right now, it's extremely difficult to draw specific conclusions from much of the microbiome data that are available from American Gut and other such companies. In fact it would be unethical to make claims unless we were really sure of being correct. It's one thing for Jack to experiment on himself through diet manipulation (and let's face it, reducing the number of candy bars and eating healthier was not exactly a risky move), but it's an entirely different issue if we want to experiment on others. However, in collaboration with Dr. Gordon Saxe at UCSD, Rob is currently exploring the effects of an anti-inflammatory diet more consistently and across a range of different conditions, so we may have more information on this soon.

Is there any way for me to track changes in my child's microbiome?

Yes, but the projects looking at this are not yet ready for consumers.

Just like the height and weight charts that we use to learn if a child's development is on track, your child's microbiome development can also be monitored. Right now, most of the work has been done in Bangladesh and Malawi, where children have very different microbiomes (and are at risk for different health conditions) than in the United States. But we are working with the Rady Children's Hospital, which is affiliated with UC San Diego, to produce exactly this kind of microbial growth chart. Once those charts exist, you'll be able to compare your child to other children, to see if they're on track and if they're at risk for any specific diseases.

Similarly, large-scale projects for inflammatory bowel disease (RISK) and type 1 diabetes (TEDDY) are currently putting together microbial growth charts for at-risk populations. Once completed, you might be able to tell if your child is developing type 1 diabetes or Crohn's disease before it happens. However, even when the data from those projects is ready, it will be difficult to add your own data to the project because different methods are being used. It will take a while before a clinical test is robust enough that you can interpret the results with confidence in the context of the larger population.

How do I use the information?

Systematic attempts to build microbial road maps that anyone can understand are still in their infancy. However, work in our labs among others is helping to provide a microbial GPS that should in future enable us to give you recommendations on how to rebalance your child's microbial health.

In general, information is provided as a list of bacterial organisms that your child has in a sample. It's like a list of your Facebook friends. It tells you what species are there and usually their relative abundance as a percentage the total number of organisms observed. Your child's report may contain species described at the level of genus. For example, the human genus is *Homo* and your child's species is *sapiens*. We call this a binomial or two-part name: *Homo sapiens*. At the level of genus, a dog (*Canis familiaris*) and a wolf (*Canis lupus*) would be indistinguishable. So if I told you that you had a *Canis* in your house, you wouldn't really know whether to be terrified or go buy kibble.

This nomenclature is a perennial problem with microbiome analysis. In the section on how to do testing, we talked about how the microbiome can be analyzed using 16S rRNA and metagenomics. The former analysis just tells us the abundance of the different genus of bacteria in your child's sample. The latter, metagenomics, can be used to make a much more refined identification. To continue our *Canis* analogy, with 16S rRNA analysis you would be confused, but with metagenomic analysis you would know what kind of animal you're dealing with.

So the method of testing is important. But, the ultimate goal of testing is to compare your results with other people. How similar is my microbiome to someone of my age, gender, and weight? Does my child's microbiome resemble that of other children with autism? These are question you can ask. The presence or abundance of a single bacteria species is rarely very useful at this stage in our understanding.

However, when we have information on how similar your child's overall microbiome is to other kids, we'll be able to make user-friendly tools you can use to ask questions about your child's profile. Are the new antibiotics or diet having an effect? Is your child at greater or lesser risk of other diseases?

Many companies are working on this approach, and it is a hot topic of research in the scientific community as well. The popularity of self-monitoring devices such as pedometers have accelerated the public's need for routine monitoring that can be used to identify pathways to health.

Microbiome monitoring is a powerful tool as well, but outside of the anecdotal stories we have provided, these tools cannot yet be built because the underlying data remain complex and difficult to interpret. We are trying to improve the data resources to ensure that we have the capacity to make these tools work the way we and everyone else wants them to. But for now, that's all in the future.

How do I know if the test results are reliable?

This is a tough question. There are least three reputable suppliers who could provide analysis (American Gut, Second Genome, uBiome). There are also hundreds of sequencing centers you can choose from that could provide a similar service if you could get hold of your own kits. There are companies such as The BioCollective (which Jack cofounded) that bank your stool just in case you need it later, and they also offer analysis services through collaboration with companies like CosmosID. There are plenty of choices, but as we noted earlier, there is still only a limited amount you can get from these data right now.

However, you should be concerned about the reliability of the data these companies will generate for you. When we use sequencing centers, including those at our own universities (UC San Diego and the University of Chicago), we always want to ensure that the data is good quality and the analysis is of the highest standard. You should demand the same. In choosing one, you'll need to rely on the company's reputation. You might want to ask if they employ the same techniques used in peer-reviewed scientific studies. Why is this important? Well, if you want to be able to interpret the findings, then it is important that the people analyzing your data use the same methods as those who did the original research.

The tools you use to do a job influence the outcome of the job. The same is true for microbiome research. The way a sample is acquired, even down to the type of swab used to sample stool, the way in which the research team extract DNA from the sample, and even the tools used to analyze the DNA, can all affect the results. In this way, molecular science (including the study of DNA) is much like cooking. We all want to make a cake, but how we go about doing it will determine how good that cake is.

Some labs may ask you to send in multiple samples, but this won't tell you much, unless there are many samples taken over a number of days. The microbial communities in your child's stool can vary tremendously from one day to the next, so a single sample is not that informative: it is much more powerful to see how the microbiome is changing over time. This variability may cause concern, but because you get different results at different times doesn't mean you have a problem. The microbiome is in flux because, like any ecosystem, it is changing as it develops. We strongly recommend samples collected over a week, or a number of weeks over a month, to capture this variability, as it is very informative as to the average composition of the microbiome and also what may be happening as the gut matures.

You should also pay attention to what different providers say about your test results. If they tell you that they're useful for research, that's probably true. If they tell you that they can be used right now to diagnose a health problem, you should be concerned. The FDA has not approved any diagnostic tests based on the microbiome. It does certify clinical labs, but only insofar as they can reproduce their findings, not whether their processes give the right answer.

Until we have sound standards based on scientific research, it's not a good idea to order tests based on user reviews. For example, with film processing you never had to worry whether the different companies were publishing scientific papers. With photos you know good results when you see them. But with clinical tests, you have no way of intuitively knowing if they're right or wrong. User reviews will not help.

The situation is similar to stem-cell therapies, where clinics are flourishing but the science is still evolving.

Conclusion:
A Few Words on Hype

We've shown you the kinds of questions we get from concerned parents and our best efforts to answer them based on current knowledge. But these sorts of exchanges can be difficult for scientists working in our field. A mother will say, "My son is really sick. I've tried everything and nothing is working. Please, please, help me! You must have something in your lab that can help!"

It can make parents feel helpless to not have answers. And it can also make a scientist feel powerful. Maybe I have partially formed answers. Maybe I can help this mother. That feeling can be intoxicating, and for some, it can lead to a kind of addiction. Such researchers will start making claims that cannot be supported by currently available data. To put it simply, they start making things up.

This abuse of authority lets down the whole science profession and can deal a major blow to public confidence in science and the scientists who are working hard to advance understanding. The origin of many of these erroneous claims comes from a place of frustration. The science is exciting and the early findings suggest a major opportunity to improve individual health. So it is very tempting to go just that one step further and say that the results support such and such a treatment.

For example, let's say a scientist identifies a bacterium in the lab that, when fed to mice, reduced symptoms of anxiety. They publish these results, go to a scientific conference and talk about the findings, maybe even do some interviews with the press. Let's say that some reporters work with the story and make a catchy headline. "Happy Bugs Can Cure Depression." Everyone reads these headlines. A few may even read the fuller story. An even smaller fraction may read the original scientific paper. In the end, many people will get the impression that science has come up with a wonder bug that can cure depression in people. In some rare cases, this cascade can be due to the scientists' own hyperbole or that of their press office. However, whatever the cause, the outcome is misinformation about what the science can do for you today.

People suffering from depression (in the case of this example) would love to have a new treatment option, especially since current treatments have major side effects and don't work for everyone. And they may start e-mailing or calling the scientist, asking how they can get this amazing new "drug" (and yes, the FDA does regulate microbes that have an effect on disease as drugs). We hope that the scientist would explain that the research is in its very early phases, that the study was only performed in animals, and that we have no real understanding as to whether this could be effective in humans. Ideally, he or she would also explain that we don't even know if the bacterium in question is safe for humans to consume, let alone whether it would be at all useful in treating depression. It's really important to remember that the same microbe has different effects in different species: for example, *Salmonella enterica* serovar Typhimurium, which causes diarrhea in people, is deadly to mice. And there are lots of examples of zoonoses, where a microbe harmless to animals is deadly when it gets into people.

In some potentially disastrous circumstances, patients may take things into their own hands, deciding that the potential risks are outweighed by their own suffering, and attempt to acquire the bacterium and start experimenting on themselves. This is not as uncommon as you might think. And the ramifications of these unsupervised and unlicensed studies can be dire, including infection, sepsis, and death.

Jack's oldest son has autism. While some of Jack's research focuses on trying to understand the connection between the microbiome and children's neurological development, including autism, if he were to uncover a potential therapy in his animal studies, he would most certainly *not* attempt to experiment on his own child. The reasons should be obvious. The science is not advanced enough to even understand if a potential treatment could be effective in humans. We do not yet know if it is safe for consumption or what the potential side effects could be. We do not know whether the treatments could have long-term consequences that we have not even considered.

Similarly, Rob's studies of the soil bacterium *Mycobacterium vaccae* with his colleagues at the University of Colorado and University College in London suggest that it has beneficial effects on analogs of social stress and depression in mice.[1] However, under no circumstances would he consider giving it to his family members who have these disorders until appropriate clinical trials in humans are conducted (although he might encourage them to enroll in such trials if they meet the technical criteria for inclusion).

Long-term consequences of any treatment always need to be considered. Imagine you took a fecal microbiome transplant to cure a *C. diff* infection in your gut. Based on our current knowledge, what might happen if the stool donor was obese? There is a small, but not insignificant likelihood that you would gain weight if you continued eating a diet high in fats and sugars. This concern is not hypothetical. One woman in Rhode Island who had a fecal transfer started to pack on pounds after the procedure. Interestingly, the donor was a family member who weighed 140 pounds at the time of the donation but who rapidly gained 30 pounds shortly after the procedure. Six months later the recipient had also gained 34 pounds, making her obese. Three years later she was still overweight at 177 pounds. To address these types of long-term consequences of fecal transplantation, the American Gastroenterological Association recently obtained funding from the National Institutes of Health to set up a nationwide registry to track all fecal transplant donors and recipients, and a biobank with openly available sequencing data from all the samples from all donors and recipients. It is being set up via our American Gut Project.

The work that we and others have done needs to be understood in the light of what it is—research. We are asking questions and findings answers, and these answers are sometimes extremely exciting and hint at what the future of medicine might hold. It seems implausible to us that microbiome-associated therapies will not play a substantial role in the future of medical treatment. However, microbiome research for the vast majority of these diseases, disorders, symptoms, and conditions is just not yet ready for clinical application. Often researchers will confuse correlation with causation. Just because two observations are linked does not mean that one causes the other. Studies end up being like the Tarot: you can tell a good story with any arbitrary combination. Much more research, and by that we mean high-quality research, needs to be done.

Microbial medicine is a very compelling idea. It's a potentially noninvasive way of rebalancing and maintaining health. That something you buy in the grocery store, be it certain types of food or probiotics, could have such a profound influence is extremely enticing. People want to have control of their health, and many are afraid of chemicals and drugs that have substantial side effects. The microbiome seems so in tune with people's understanding of their health. All the little twitches and symptoms that come and go suddenly have an explanation and strategies to apply for making it all better.

We wish it were so simple.

As with all diseases and treatments, it's essential that we determine whether the treatment is effective, what its side effects are, and whether it works in a broad enough population. We are moving into a world of precision medicine, whereby these characteristics may be evaluated in individual people, so that treatments can be fine-tuned to their needs. The microbiome can play a substantial role in helping doctors to identify a disease and, potentially, offer novel avenues for treatment. But this will always be in collaboration with all other treatment options.

A great example comes from the world of cancer. One of Jack's colleagues at University of Chicago, Thomas Gajewski, identified certain bacteria that when fed to mice can improve the efficacy of a treatment for melanoma.[2] The therapy uses drugs that help activate the immune system to fight this deadly skin cancer, and doctors have been able to significantly improve outcomes for many patients. However, many others do not respond. Dr. Gajewski's work with mice showed that the therapy worked better when combined with a probiotic bacterium (*Bacteroides fragilis*). This meant that more mice showed a reduction in tumor size and growth when taking the combined therapy (immune blockade and probiotic) than when taking the immune blockade therapy alone.

Obviously, some melanoma patients would be interested in this new combination as a better way to go. However, as

Dr Gajewski often stresses, this therapy has only been shown to work in mice. But that has not stopped people from trying to develop it. A company called Evelo LLC has recently invested $30 million in this combined therapy, hoping to get to a stage where human trials can be started.

Clinical trials are hard. For example, Seres Therapeutics tried to reduce the uncertainty inherent in fecal transplants for C. *diff* by using a cocktail of individual bacteria isolated from stool. All were manufactured according to FDA standards for drugs. The phase 1 safety trial was very promising, with high rates of success comparable to a natural fecal transplant. However, in phase 2 (for efficacy), they changed the preparation method and the target population, and their "microbial drug" didn't work any better than a placebo. They are analyzing the data to find out why, but this reinforces the point that even if a drug (or microbe) works in one specific population that doesn't mean it will work for you. Even products with the best theoretical basis for working don't always succeed when put into practice. Of course this isn't limited to microbes: the hormone leptin, which is amazing at slimming down fat mice, doesn't work at all in humans except for a tiny fraction of the population who have a very specific and rare genetic defect.

Microbiome-based therapeutics, whether alone or in combination with other therapies are extremely exciting, but we must temper the excitement and not get carried away and give people either false hope or bad ideas about self-experimentation. We need to be careful about the messages we put out there. But we also need to be inventive and creative, and build the next generation of scientific advances by dreaming about what could be possible.

This book contains the current state of the art for microbiome science. We focus on the actual, credible evidence that supports potential therapies or existing therapies for treating disease. We hope that some the evidence and advice we provide will help parents navigate this confusing but enticing field.

In parting, we want you to consider one thing about the evidence you use in making decisions for your child. Use critical thinking in making that decision. Leave your biases at the door. Don't go looking for data or conclusions that support your expectations. Try to read news or scientific articles without preconceived notions of what you expect to find. Try to read the full news article, even if you don't agree with the title or headline. Explore the background if you can. Look for confirming evidence on web sites like clinicaltrials.gov or at university hospitals or internationally respected clinics. And ask yourself two simple questions: does this research justify how it was interpreted? And does it have any relevance for my concerns? That is, is there anything here that you can use to help you in looking after your child? If you have doubts, you should trust your feelings.

In the end, you are the parent. You are the person responsible for making the decision, and you have to own that responsibility, come good or bad outcomes. We are both parents, and we know that we often make mistakes. We are sure our parents did just as well as we did. But if your child has a condition that is dealt with in this book, we hope the information will prove useful.

Good luck!

Acknowledgments

First of all, we want to thank the people who convinced us that this book needed to be written, including all those who asked us questions at every meeting we have ever attended. This constant thirst for understanding has been one of the driving forces behind our desire to encapsulate the science behind the buzz of the microbiome.

We would also like to thank Ed Yong, who listened to all of our questions about publishing and writing a book, and to Neil Shubin, who was peppered with questions about what it was like as a scientist to publish and capture the correct angle. Ed and Neil also helped us, albeit indirectly, to choose our agent, James Levine, who immediately grasped the ideas we wanted to convey. He helped us explore the landscape of what to expect from both publishers and readers and showed us how working with Sandra Blakeslee would lead to a better book. If we had worked with Sandra as ghostwriter, we would be expounding more specifically here about her contributions. Instead, we felt immediately that we were a team that contributed equally to the text in many ways. We are grateful to her for working closely with us, ensuring that the science is both accurate and accessible.

We would like to especially thank Jack's wife, Katharine Gilbert, and Rob's partner, Amanda Birmingham, for believing in this crazy idea and for lending invaluable support and advice on the book's contents. We are also indebted to our parents, Hilary and Anthony Gilbert and Drs. John and Allison Knight, who read early drafts and kindly refrained from commenting on our punctuation.

We also want to thank the many people who contributed ideas for this book or commented on drafts, including Erin Lane, Brian and Nadda Kwilosz, Dr. John Alverdy, Alison Vrbanac, Dr. Nicole Scott, Dr. Jairam, K. P. Vanamala, Dr. Chris Callewaert, Dr. Marty Blaser, Dr. Maria Gloria Dominguez-Bello, Hannes Holste, Dr. Jae Kim, Dr. Gabriel Haddad, Dr. Emily Lukacz, Dr. Linda Brubaker, Dr. Marie-Claire Arrieta, Dr. Fernando Perez, Dr. Eugene Chang, Martha Carlin, Dr. Daniel van der Lelie, and Dr. Rick Stevens. We would also like to thank the hundreds of collaborators and colleagues whose ideas we hope we have reflected accurately in this work.

Finally, we want to thank the funding agencies and our institutions (Argonne National Laboratory, University of Chicago, University of California at San Diego, and the Marine Biological Laboratory) for supporting the science and investigations that have led to the evidence presented here.

Importantly, we are keen to thank all the participants in all the clinical trials who so willingly gave their time, energy, and samples to make the research possible. By donating your poop, you have helped change the world.

Notes

Chapter 1: The Microbiome

1. Weiss, M. C., et al. (2016). The physiology and habitat of the last universal common ancestor. *Nat. Microbiol., 1,* 16116.
2. Lennon, J. T., & Locey, K. J. (2016). The underestimation of global microbial diversity. *mBio, 7,* e01298–16.

Chapter 2: The Human Microbiome

1. Sender, R., Fuchs, S., & Milo, R. (2016). Revised estimates for the number of human and bacteria cells in the body. *PLoS Biol., 14,* e1002533.

Chapter 3: Pregnancy

1. Rizzo, A., et al. (2015). Lactobacillus crispatus mediates anti-inflammatory cytokine interleukin-10 induction in response to Chlamydia trachomatis infection in vitro. *Int. J. Med. Microbiol., 305,* 815–827.
2. Van Oostrum, N., De Sutter, P., Meys, J., & Verstraelen, H. (2013). Risks associated with bacterial vaginosis in infertility patients: a systematic review and meta-analysis. *Hum. Reprod. Oxf. Engl., 28,* 1809–1815.
3. Weng, S.-L., et al. (2014). Bacterial communities in semen from men of infertile couples: metagenomic sequencing reveals relationships of seminal microbiota to semen quality. *PloS One, 9,* e110152.
4. Lax, S., et al. (2014). Longitudinal analysis of microbial interaction between humans and the indoor environment. *Science, 345,* 1048–1052.
5. Song, S. J., et al. (2013). Cohabiting family members share microbiota with one another and with their dogs. *eLife, 2,* e00458.
6. Ibid.
7. Nakano, K., et al. (2009). Detection of oral bacteria in cardiovascular specimens. *Oral Microbiol. Immunol., 24,* 64–68.

8. Madianos, P. N., Bobetsis, Y. A., & Offenbacher, S. (2013). Adverse pregnancy outcomes (APOs) and periodontal disease: pathogenic mechanisms. *J. Periodontol., 84,* S170–S180; Bobetsis, Y. A., Barros, S. P., & Offenbacher, S. (2006). Exploring the relationship between periodontal disease and pregnancy complications. *J. Am. Dent. Assoc., 137,* Suppl, 7S–13S.

9. Durand, R., Gunselman, E. L., Hodges, J. S., Diangelis, A. J., & Michalowicz, B. S. (2009). A pilot study of the association between cariogenic oral bacteria and preterm birth. *Oral Dis., 15,* 400–406.

10. Pozo, E., et al. (2016). Preterm birth and/or low birth weight are associated with periodontal disease and the increased placental immunohistochemical expression of inflammatory markers. *Histol. Histopathol., 31,* 231–237.

11. Corbella, S., Taschieri, S., Francetti, L., De Siena, F., & Del Fabbro, M. (2012). Periodontal disease as a risk factor for adverse pregnancy outcomes: a systematic review and meta-analysis of case-control studies. *Odontology, 100,* 232–240.

12. Smith-Spangler, C., et al. (2012). Are organic foods safer or healthier than conventional alternatives? A systematic review. *Ann. Intern. Med., 157,* 348.

13. Alcock, I., White, M. P., Wheeler, B. W., Fleming, L. E., & Depledge, M. H. (2014). Longitudinal effects on mental health of moving to greener and less green urban areas. *Environ. Sci. Technol., 48,* 1247–1255.

14. Breton, J., et al. (2016). Gut commensal E. coli proteins activate host satiety pathways following nutrient-induced bacterial growth. *Cell Metab., 23,* 324–334.

15. Rezzi, S., et al. (2007). Human metabolic phenotypes link directly to specific dietary preferences in healthy individuals. *J. Proteome Res., 6,* 4469–4477.

16. Leone, V., et al. (2015). Effects of diurnal variation of gut microbes and high-fat feeding on host circadian clock function and metabolism. *Cell Host Microbe, 17,* 681–689.

17. Santacruz, A., et al. (2010). Gut microbiota composition is associated with body weight, weight gain and biochemical parameters in pregnant women. *Br. J. Nutr., 104,* 83–92.

18. Bajaj, K., & Gross, S. J. (2015). The genetics of diabetic pregnancy. *Best Pract. Res. Clin. Obstet. Gynaecol., 29,* 102–109.

19. Fuller, M., et al. (2015). The short-chain fatty acid receptor, FFA2, contributes to gestational glucose homeostasis. *Am. J. Physiol. Endocrinol. Metab., 309,* E840–E851.

20. Allen, J. M., et al. (2015). Voluntary and forced exercise differentially alters the gut microbiome in C57BL/6J mice. *J. Appl. Physiol. Bethesda Md (1985), 118,* 1059–1066.

21. Kang, S. S., et al. (2014). Diet and exercise orthogonally alter the gut microbiome and reveal independent associations with anxiety and cognition. *Mol. Neurodegener., 9,* 36.

22. Tibaldi, C., et al. (2016). Maternal risk factors for abnormal vaginal flora during pregnancy. *Int. J. Gynaecol. Obstet. Off. Organ Int. Fed. Gynaecol. Obstet., 133,* 89–93; Donders, G. G. G. (2015). Reducing infection-related preterm birth. *BJOG Int. J. Obstet. Gynaecol., 122,* 219; Newton, E. R., Piper, J., & Peairs, W. (1997). Bacterial vaginosis and intraamniotic infection. *Am. J. Obstet. Gynecol., 176,* 672–677.

23. Prince, A. L., et al. (2016). The placental membrane microbiome is altered among subjects with spontaneous preterm birth with and without chorioamnionitis. *Am. J. Obstet. Gynecol., 214,* 627.e1–627.e16.

24. Abramovici, A., et al. (2015). Quantitative polymerase chain reaction to assess response to treatment of bacterial vaginosis and risk of preterm birth. *Am. J. Perinatol., 32,* 1119–1125.

25. Yang, S., et al. (2015). Is there a role for probiotics in the prevention of preterm birth? *Front. Immunol., 6,* 62; Yang, S., et al. (2014). Probiotic Lactobacillus rhamnosus GR-1 supernatant prevents lipopolysaccharide-induced preterm birth and reduces inflammation in pregnant CD-1 mice. *Am. J. Obstet. Gynecol., 211,* 44.e1–44.e12.

26. Bierne, H., et al. (2012). Activation of type III interferon genes by pathogenic bacteria in infected epithelial cells and mouse placenta. *PloS One, 7,* e39080.

27. Lemas, D. J., et al. (2016). Exploring the contribution of maternal antibiotics and breastfeeding to development of the infant microbiome and pediatric obesity. *Semin. Fetal. Neonatal Med., 21,* 406–409.

28. Stokholm, J., et al. (2014). Antibiotic use during pregnancy alters the commensal vaginal microbiota. *Clin. Microbiol. Infect. Off. Publ. Eur. Soc. Clin. Microbiol. Infect. Dis., 20,* 629–635.

29. Mueller, N. T., et al. (2015). Prenatal exposure to antibiotics, cesarean section and risk of childhood obesity. *Int. J. Obes. 2005, 39,* 665–670.

30. Kuperman, A. A., & Koren, O. (2016). Antibiotic use during pregnancy: How bad is it? *BMC Med., 14,* 91.

31. Tormo-Badia, N., et al. (2014). Antibiotic treatment of pregnant non-obese diabetic mice leads to altered gut microbiota and intestinal immunological changes in the offspring. *Scand. J. Immunol., 80,* 250–260; Ledger, W. J., & Blaser, M. J. (2013). Are we using too many antibiotics during pregnancy? *BJOG Int. J. Obstet. Gynaecol., 120,* 1450–1452; Metsälä, J., et al. (2013). Mother's and offspring's use of antibiotics and infant allergy to cow's milk. *Epidemiol. Camb. Mass, 24,* 303–309; Atladóttir, H. Ó., Henriksen, T. B., Schendel, D.

E., & Parner, E. T. (2012). Autism after infection, febrile episodes, and antibiotic use during pregnancy: An exploratory study. *Pediatrics, 130,* e1447–1454; Stensballe, L. G., Simonsen, J., Jensen, S. M., Bønnelykke, K., & Bisgaard, H. (2013). Use of antibiotics during pregnancy increases the risk of asthma in early childhood. *J. Pediatr., 162,* 832–838.e3.

32. Stensballe, L. G., Simonsen, J., Jensen, S. M., Bønnelykke, K., & Bisgaard, H. (2013). Use of antibiotics during pregnancy increases the risk of asthma in early childhood. *J. Pediatr., 162,* 832–838.e3; Kaplan, Y. C., Keskin-Arslan, E., Acar, S., & Sozmen, K. (2016). Prenatal selective serotonin reuptake inhibitor use and the risk of autism spectrum disorder in children: A systematic review and meta-analysis. *Reprod. Toxicol. Elmsford N, 66,* 31–43; Alwan, S., Friedman, J. M., & Chambers, C. (2016). Safety of selective serotonin reuptake inhibitors in pregnancy: A review of current evidence. *CNS Drugs, 30,* 499–515; Ross, L. E., et al. (2013). Selected pregnancy and delivery outcomes after exposure to antidepressant medication: a systematic review and meta-analysis. *JAMA Psychiatry, 70,* 436–443; El Marroun, H., et al. (2012). Maternal use of selective serotonin reuptake inhibitors, fetal growth, and risk of adverse birth outcomes. *Arch. Gen. Psychiatry, 69,* 706–714.

Chapter 4: Birth

1. Hutton, E. K., et al. (2016). Outcomes associated with planned place of birth among women with low-risk pregnancies. *CMAJ Can. Med. Assoc. J. J. Assoc. Medicale Can., 188,* E80–E90.

2. Illuzzi, J. L., Stapleton, S. R., & Rathbun, L. (2015). Early and total neonatal mortality in relation to birth setting in the United States, 2006–2009. *Am. J. Obstet. Gynecol., 212,* 250.

3. Cheyney, M., et al. (2014). Outcomes of care for 16,924 planned home births in the United States: The Midwives Alliance of North America Statistics Project, 2004 to 2009. *J. Midwifery Women's Health, 59,* 17–27.

4. Janssen, P. A., et al. (2002). Outcomes of planned home births versus planned hospital births after regulation of midwifery in British Columbia. *CMAJ Can. Med. Assoc. J. J. Assoc. Medicale Can., 166,* 315–323.

5. Hutton, E. K., Reitsma, A., Thorpe, J., Brunton, G., & Kaufman, K. (2014). Protocol: Systematic review and meta-analyses of birth outcomes for women who intend at the onset of labour to give birth at home compared to women of low obstetrical risk who intend to give birth in hospital. *Syst. Rev., 3,* 55.

6. Illuzzi, J. L., Stapleton, S. R., & Rathbun, L. (2015). Early and total neonatal mortality in relation to birth setting in the United States, 2006–2009. *Am. J. Obstet. Gynecol., 212,* 250.

7. Aagaard, K., et al. (2014). The placenta harbors a unique microbiome. *Sci. Transl. Med., 6,* 237ra65; Lauder, A. P., et al. (2016). Comparison of placenta samples with contamination controls does not provide evidence for a distinct placenta microbiota. *Microbiome, 4,* 29.

8. Dominguez-Bello, M. G., et al. (2010). Delivery mode shapes the acquisition and structure of the initial microbiota across multiple body habitats in newborns. *Proc. Natl. Acad. Sci. U.S.A., 107,* 11971–11975.

9. Dominguez-Bello, M. G., et al. (2016). Partial restoration of the microbiota of cesarean-born infants via vaginal microbial transfer. *Nat. Med., 22* (3), 250–253, doi:10.1038/nm.4039.

10. Portela, D. S., Vieira, T. O., Matos, S. M., de Oliveira, N. F., & Vieira, G. O. (2015). Maternal obesity, environmental factors, cesarean delivery and breastfeeding as determinants of overweight and obesity in children: Results from a cohort. *BMC Pregnancy Childbirth, 15,* 94; Pei, Z., et al. (2014). Cesarean delivery and risk of childhood obesity. *J. Pediatr., 164,* 1068–1073.e2; Huh, S. Y., et al. (2012). Delivery by caesarean section and risk of obesity in preschool age children: A prospective cohort study. *Arch. Dis. Child., 97,* 610–616; Blustein, J., et al. (2013). Association of caesarean delivery with child adiposity from age 6 weeks to 15 years. *Int. J. Obes. 2005, 37,* 900–906.

11. Henningsson, A., Nyström, B., & Tunnell, R. (1981). Bathing or washing babies after birth? *Lancet Lond. Engl., 2,* 1401–1403.

12. Shulak, B. (1963). The antibacterial action of vernix caseosa. *Harper Hosp. Bull., 21,* 111–117; Jha, A. K., Baliga, S., Kumar, H. H., Rangnekar, A., & Baliga, B. S. (2015). Is there a preventive role for vernix caseosa? An invitro study. *J. Clin. Diagn. Res., 9,* SC13–16.

13. Warner, B. B., et al. (2016). Gut bacteria dysbiosis and necrotising enterocolitis in very low birthweight infants: A prospective case-control study. *Lancet Lond. Engl., 387,* 1928–1936.

14. McMurtry, V. E., et al. (2015). Bacterial diversity and clostridia abundance decrease with increasing severity of necrotizing enterocolitis. *Microbiome, 3,* 11.

15. Niemarkt, H. J., et al. (2015). Necrotizing enterocolitis: A clinical review on diagnostic biomarkers and the role of the intestinal microbiota. *Inflamm. Bowel Dis., 21,* 436–444.

16. Underwood, M. A. (2016). Impact of probiotics on necrotizing enterocolitis. *Semin. Perinatol.* doi:10.1053/j.semperi.2016.09.017.

17. Penders, J., et al. (2014). New insights into the hygiene hypothesis in allergic diseases: Mediation of sibling and birth mode effects by the gut microbiota. *Gut Microbes, 5,* 239–244.

18. Penders, J., et al. (2013). Establishment of the intestinal microbiota and its role for atopic dermatitis in early childhood. *J. Allergy Clin. Immunol., 132,* 601–607.e8.

19. Human Microbiome Project Consortium. (2012). Structure, function and diversity of the healthy human microbiome. *Nature, 486,* 207–214.

20. Ibid.

21. Zozaya, M., et al. (2016). Bacterial communities in penile skin, male urethra, and vaginas of heterosexual couples with and without bacterial vaginosis. *Microbiome, 4,* 16.

22. Song, S. J., et al. (2013). Cohabiting family members share microbiota with one another and with their dogs. *eLife, 2,* e00458; Yatsunenko, T., et al. (2012). Human gut microbiome viewed across age and geography. *Nature.* doi:10.1038/nature11053.

Chapter 5: Breast-Feeding

1. Kramer, M. S., et al. (2007). Effects of prolonged and exclusive breastfeeding on child height, weight, adiposity, and blood pressure at age 6.5 y: Evidence from a large randomized trial. *Am. J. Clin. Nutr., 86,* 1717–1721.

2. Sela, D. A., et al. (2008). The genome sequence of Bifidobacterium longum subsp. infantis reveals adaptations for milk utilization within the infant microbiome. *Proc. Natl. Acad. Sci. U.S.A., 105,* 18964–18969; Bode, L. (2009). Human milk oligosaccharides: Prebiotics and beyond. *Nutr. Rev., 67* Suppl 2, S183–191; Yu, Z.-T., et al. (2013). The principal fucosylated oligosaccharides of human milk exhibit prebiotic properties on cultured infant microbiota. *Glycobiology, 23,* 169–177.

3. Sela, D. A., et al. (2008). The genome sequence of Bifidobacterium longum subsp. infantis reveals adaptations for milk utilization within the infant microbiome. *Proc. Natl. Acad. Sci. U.S.A., 105,* 18964–18969.

4. Charbonneau, M. R., et al. (2016). Sialylated milk oligosaccharides promote microbiota-dependent growth in models of infant undernutrition. *Cell, 164,* 859–871.

5. Bode, L. (2009). Human milk oligosaccharides: Prebiotics and beyond. *Nutr. Rev., 67* Suppl 2, S183–S191.

6. Goldsmith, A. J., et al. (2016). Formula and breast feeding in infant food allergy: A population-based study. *J. Paediatr. Child Health, 52,* 377–384.

7. Bloom, B. T. (2016). Safety of donor milk: A brief report. *J. Perinatol. Off. J. Calif. Perinat. Assoc., 36,* 392–393.

8. Bravi, F., et al. (2016). Impact of maternal nutrition on breast-milk composition: A systematic review. *Am. J. Clin. Nutr., 104,* 646–662.

9. Grote, V., et al. (2016). Breast milk composition and infant nutrient intakes during the first 12 months of life. *Eur. J. Clin. Nutr., 70,* 250–256.

10. Prentice, A. M., et al. (1980). Dietary supplementation of Gambian nursing mothers and lactational performance. *The Lancet, 316,* 886–888.

11. Makrides, M., Neumann, M. A., & Gibson, R. A. (1996). Effect of maternal docosahexaenoic acid (DHA) supplementation on breast milk composition. *Eur. J. Clin. Nutr., 50,* 352–357.

12. Dunstan, J. A., et al. (2004). The effect of supplementation with fish oil during pregnancy on breast milk immunoglobulin A, soluble CD14, cytokine levels and fatty acid composition. *Clin. Exp. Allergy J. Br. Soc. Allergy Clin. Immunol., 34,* 1237–1242.

13. Chung, A. M., Reed, M. D., & Blumer, J. L. (2002). Antibiotics and breast-feeding: A critical review of the literature. *Paediatr. Drugs, 4,* 817–837.

14. Newton, E. R., & Hale, T. W. (2015). Drugs in breast milk. *Clin. Obstet. Gynecol., 58,* 868–884.

15. Dubois, N. E., & Gregory, K. E. (2016). Characterizing the intestinal microbiome in infantile colic: Findings based on an integrative review of the literature. *Biol. Res. Nurs., 18,* 307–315.

16. De Weerth, C., Fuentes, S., Puylaert, P., & de Vos, W. M. (2013). Intestinal microbiota of infants with colic: Development and specific signatures. *Pediatrics, 131,* e550–558.

17. Indrio, F., et al. (2014). Prophylactic use of a probiotic in the prevention of colic, regurgitation, and functional constipation: A randomized clinical trial. *JAMA Pediatr., 168,* 228–233.

Chapter 6: Antibiotics

1. Dargaville, P. A., Copnell, B., & Australian and New Zealand Neonatal Network. (2006). The epidemiology of meconium aspiration syndrome: Incidence, risk factors, therapies, and outcome. *Pediatrics, 117,* 1712–1721.

2. Lee, J., et al. (2016). Meconium aspiration syndrome: A role for fetal systemic inflammation. *Am. J. Obstet. Gynecol., 214,* 366.e1–9.

3. Zloto, O., et al. (2016). Ophthalmia neonatorum treatment and prophylaxis: IPOSC global study. *Graefes Arch. Clin. Exp. Ophthalmol., 254,* 577–582.

4. Theriot, C. M., et al. (2014). Antibiotic-induced shifts in the mouse gut microbiome and metabolome increase susceptibility to Clostridium difficile infection. *Nat. Commun., 5,* 3114.

5. Dethlefsen, L., & Relman, D. A. (2011). Incomplete recovery and individualized responses of the human distal gut microbiota to repeated antibiotic perturbation. *Proc. Natl. Acad. Sci. U.S.A., 108* Suppl 1, 4554–4561.

6. Cox, L. M., & Blaser, M. J. (2015). Antibiotics in early life and obesity. *Nat. Rev. Endocrinol., 11,* 182–190.

7. Benjamin Neelon, S. E., et al. (2015). Early child care and obesity at 12 months of age in the Danish National Birth Cohort. *Int. J. Obes. 2005, 39,* 33–38.

8. Gerber, J. S., et al. (2016). Antibiotic exposure during the first 6 months of life and weight gain during childhood. *JAMA, 315,* 1258.

9. Cho, I., et al. (2012). Antibiotics in early life alter the murine colonic microbiome and adiposity. *Nature, 488,* 621–626.

Chapter 7: Probiotics

1. Sood, A., et al. (2009). The probiotic preparation, VSL#3 induces remission in patients with mild-to-moderately active ulcerative colitis. *Clin. Gastroenterol. Hepatol., 7,* 1202–1209, 1209.e1; Gaudier, E., Michel, C., Segain, J.-P., Cherbut, C., & Hoebler, C. (2005). The VSL#3 probiotic mixture modifies microflora but does not heal chronic dextran-sodium sulfate-induced colitis or reinforce the mucus barrier in mice. *J. Nutr., 135,* 2753–2761; Kim, H. J., et al. (2005). A randomized controlled trial of a probiotic combination VSL#3 and placebo in irritable bowel syndrome with bloating. *Neurogastroenterol. Motil., 17,* 687–696; Loguercio, C., et al. (2005). Beneficial effects of a probiotic VSL#3 on parameters of liver dysfunction in chronic liver diseases. *J. Clin. Gastroenterol., 39,* 540–543; Kim, H. J., et al. (2003). A randomized controlled trial of a probiotic, VSL#3, on gut transit and symptoms in diarrhoea-predominant irritable bowel syndrome. *Aliment. Pharmacol. Ther., 17,* 895–904.

2. Matsuzaki, T., & Chin, J. (2000). Modulating immune responses with probiotic bacteria. *Immunol. Cell Biol., 78,* 67–73.

3. Berni Canani, R., et al. (2016). Lactobacillus rhamnosus GG-supplemented formula expands butyrate-producing bacterial strains in food allergic infants. *ISME J., 10,* 742–750.

4. Tang, M. L. K., et al. (2015). Administration of a probiotic with peanut oral immunotherapy: A randomized trial. *J. Allergy Clin. Immunol., 135,* 737–744.e8.

5. Zuccotti, G., et al. (2015). Probiotics for prevention of atopic diseases in infants: Systematic review and meta-analysis. *Allergy, 70,* 1356–1371.

6. Allen, S. J., et al. (2014). Probiotics in the prevention of eczema: A randomised controlled trial. *Arch. Dis. Child., 99,* 1014–1019.

7. Thomas, C. L., & Fernández-Peñas, P. (2016). The microbiome and atopic eczema: More than skin deep. *Australas. J. Dermatol.* doi:10.1111/ajd.12435.

8. Salarkia, N., Ghadamli, L., Zaeri, F., & Sabaghian Rad, L. (2013). Effects of probiotic yogurt on performance, respiratory and digestive systems of young adult female endurance swimmers: A randomized controlled trial. *Med. J. Islam. Repub. Iran, 27,* 141–146.

9. Di Pierro, F., Di Pasquale, D., & Di Cicco, M. (2015). Oral use of Streptococcus salivarius K12 in children with secretory otitis media: Preliminary results of a pilot, uncontrolled study. *Int. J. Gen. Med., 8,* 303–308.

10. Dominguez-Bello, M. G., & Blaser, M. J. (2008). Do you have a probiotic in your future? *Microbes Infect., 10,* 1072–1076.

11. Szajewska, H., & Mrukowicz, J. Z. (2001). Probiotics in the treatment and prevention of acute infectious diarrhea in infants and children: A systematic review of published randomized, double-blind, placebo-controlled trials. *J. Pediatr. Gastroenterol. Nutr., 33* Suppl 2, S17–S25.

12. Mohsin, M., Guenther, S., Schierack, P., Tedin, K., & Wieler, L. H. (2015). Probiotic Escherichia coli Nissle 1917 reduces growth, Shiga toxin expression, release and thus cytotoxicity of enterohemorrhagic Escherichia coli. *Int. J. Med. Microbiol., 305,* 20–26.

13. Sazawal, S., et al. (2006). Efficacy of probiotics in prevention of acute diarrhoea: A meta-analysis of masked, randomised, placebo-controlled trials. *Lancet Infect. Dis., 6,* 374–382.

14. Slattery, J., MacFabe, D. F., & Frye, R. E. (2016). The significance of the enteric microbiome on the development of childhood disease: A review of prebiotic and probiotic therapies in disorders of childhood. *Clin. Med. Insights Pediatr., 10,* 91–107.

15. McFadden, R.-M. T., et al. (2015). The role of curcumin in modulating colonic microbiota during colitis and colon cancer prevention. *Inflamm. Bowel Dis., 21,* 2483–2494.

16. Cao, Y., et al. (2016). Modulation of gut microbiota by berberine improves steatohepatitis in high-fat diet-fed BALB/C Mice. *Arch. Iran. Med., 19,* 197–203.

Chapter 8: Child Diet

1. Vandeputte, D., et al. (2016). Stool consistency is strongly associated with gut microbiota richness and composition, enterotypes and bacterial growth rates. *Gut, 65,* 57–62.

2. Franciscovich, A., et al. (2015). PoopMD, a mobile health application, accurately identifies infant acholic stools. *PLoS One, 10,* e0132270.

3. Pelto, G. H., Zhang, Y., & Habicht, J.-P. (2010). Premastication: The second arm of infant and young child feeding for health and survival? *Matern. Child. Nutr., 6,* 4–18.

4. Lack, G., & Penagos, M. (2011). Early feeding practices and development of food allergies. *Nestle Nutr. Workshop Ser. Paediatr. Programme, 68,* 169–183; discussion 183–186.

5. Blanton, L. V., Barratt, M. J., Charbonneau, M. R., Ahmed, T., & Gordon, J. I. (2016). Childhood undernutrition, the gut microbiota, and microbiota-directed therapeutics. *Science, 352,* 1533.

6. Smith, M. I., et al. (2013). Gut microbiomes of Malawian twin pairs discordant for kwashiorkor. *Science, 339,* 548–554.

7. Du Toit, G., et al. (2015). Randomized trial of peanut consumption in infants at risk for peanut allergy. *N. Engl. J. Med., 372,* 803–813.

8. Rachid, R., & Chatila, T. A. (2016). The role of the gut microbiota in food allergy. *Curr. Opin. Pediatr., 28,* 748–753.

9. Clemente, J. C., et al. (2015). The microbiome of uncontacted Amerindians. *Sci. Adv., 1,* e1500183–e1500183; Dominguez-Bello, M. G., et al. (2016). Ethics of exploring the microbiome of native peoples. *Nat. Microbiol., 1,* 16097; Turroni, S., et al. (2016). Fecal metabolome of the Hadza hunter-gatherers: A host-microbiome integrative view. *Sci. Rep., 6,* 32826.

10. Leone, V., et al. (2015). Effects of diurnal variation of gut microbes and high-fat feeding on host circadian clock function and metabolism. *Cell Host Microbe, 17,* 681–689.

11. Dewhirst, F. E. (2016). The oral microbiome: Critical for understanding oral health and disease. *J. Calif. Dent. Assoc., 44,* 409–410.

12. Thaiss, C. A., et al. (2016). Persistent microbiome alterations modulate the rate of post-dieting weight regain. *Nature.* doi:10.1038/nature20796.

13. Zhang, C., et al. (2015). Dietary modulation of gut microbiota contributes to alleviation of both genetic and simple obesity in children. *EBioMedicine, 2,* 968–984.

14. Smith-Spangler, C., et al. (2012). Are organic foods safer or healthier than conventional alternatives? A systematic review. *Ann. Intern. Med., 157,* 348.

15. Holme, F., et al. (2016). The role of diet in children's exposure to organophosphate pesticides. *Environ. Res., 147,* 133–140.

16. Schrödl, W., et al. (2014). Possible effects of glyphosate on mucorales abundance in the rumen of dairy cows in Germany. *Curr. Microbiol., 69,* 817–823.

17. Suez, J., et al. (2014). Artificial sweeteners induce glucose intolerance by altering the gut microbiota. *Nature, 514,* 181–186.

18. Giulivo, M., Lopez de Alda, M., Capri, E., & Barceló, D. (2016). Human exposure to endocrine disrupting compounds: Their role in reproductive systems, metabolic syndrome and breast cancer. A review. *Environ. Res., 151,* 251–264.

19. Oishi, K., et al. (2008). Effect of probiotics, Bifidobacterium breve and Lactobacillus casei, on bisphenol A exposure in rats. *Biosci. Biotechnol. Biochem., 72,* 1409–1415.

Chapter 9: Child Gut

1. Faith, J. J., et al. (2013). The long-term stability of the human gut microbiota. *Science, 341,* 1237439.

2. Dominguez-Bello, M. G., et al. (2010). Delivery mode shapes the acquisition and structure of the initial microbiota across multiple body habitats in newborns. *Proc. Natl. Acad. Sci. U.S.A., 107,* 11971–11975.

3. Bäckhed, F., et al. (2015). Dynamics and stabilization of the human gut microbiome during the first year of life. *Cell Host Microbe, 17,* 852.

4. Koenig, J. E., et al. (2011). Succession of microbial consortia in the developing infant gut microbiome. *Proc. Natl. Acad. Sci. U.S.A., 108* Suppl 1, 4578–4585.

5. Faith, J. J., et al. (2013). The long-term stability of the human gut microbiota. *Science, 341,* 1237439.

6. Palm, N. W., et al. (2014). Immunoglobulin A coating identifies colitogenic bacteria in inflammatory bowel disease. *Cell, 158,* 1000–1010.

7. Barr, J. J., et al. (2013). Bacteriophage adhering to mucus provide a non-host-derived immunity. *Proc. Natl. Acad. Sci. U.S.A., 110,* 10771–10776.

8. Vandeputte, D., et al. (2016). Stool consistency is strongly associated with gut microbiota richness and composition, enterotypes and bacterial growth rates. *Gut, 65,* 57–62.

9. Mello, C. S., et al. (2016). Gut microbiota differences in children from distinct socioeconomic levels living in the same urban area in Brazil. *J. Pediatr. Gastroenterol. Nutr., 63,* 460–465.

10. Yatsunenko, T., et al. (2012). Human gut microbiome viewed across age and geography. *Nature.* doi:10.1038/nature11053.

11. Goodrich, J. K., et al. (2014). Human genetics shape the gut microbiome. *Cell, 159,* 789–799.

12. Braun-Fahrländer, C., et al. (2002). Environmental exposure to endotoxin and its relation to asthma in school-age children. *N. Engl. J. Med.*, *347*, 869–877; Riedler, J., et al. (2001). Exposure to farming in early life and development of asthma and allergy: A cross-sectional survey. *Lancet Lond. Engl.*, *358*, 1129–1133.
13. Ibid.

Chapter 10: Depression

1. Kennedy, P. J., Cryan, J. F., Dinan, T. G., & Clarke, G. (2017). Kynurenine pathway metabolism and the microbiota-gut-brain axis. *Neuropharmacology*, *112*, 399–412.
2. Bravo, J. A., et al. (2012). Communication between gastrointestinal bacteria and the nervous system. *Curr. Opin. Pharmacol.*, *12*, 667–672.
3. Messaoudi, M., et al. (2011). Assessment of psychotropic-like properties of a probiotic formulation (Lactobacillus helveticus R0052 and Bifidobacterium longum R0175) in rats and human subjects. *Br. J. Nutr.*, *105*, 755–764.
4. Gacias, M., et al. (2016). Microbiota-driven transcriptional changes in prefrontal cortex override genetic differences in social behavior. *eLife*, *5*:e13442; Hoban, A. E., et al. (2016). Regulation of prefrontal cortex myelination by the microbiota. *Transl. Psychiatry*, *6*, e774; Braniste, V., et al. (2014). The gut microbiota influences blood-brain barrier permeability in mice. *Sci. Transl. Med.*, *6*, 263ra158; Janik, R., et al. (2016). Magnetic resonance spectroscopy reveals oral Lactobacillus promotion of increases in brain GABA, N-acetyl aspartate and glutamate. *NeuroImage*, *125*, 988–995; Sampson, T. R., et al. (2016). Gut microbiota regulate motor deficits and neuroinflammation in a model of Parkinson's disease. *Cell*, *167*, 1469–1480.e12; Mitew, S., Kirkcaldie, M. T. K., Dickson, T. C., & Vickers, J. C. (2013). Altered synapses and gliotransmission in Alzheimer's disease and AD model mice. *Neurobiol. Aging*, *34*, 2341–2351; Bravo, J. A., et al. (2011). Ingestion of Lactobacillus strain regulates emotional behavior and central GABA receptor expression in a mouse via the vagus nerve. *Proc. Natl. Acad. Sci.*, *108*, 16050–16055.
5. Zheng, P., et al. (2016). Gut microbiome remodeling induces depressive-like behaviors through a pathway mediated by the host's metabolism. *Mol. Psychiatry*, *21*, 786–796.

Chapter 11: Vaccines

1. "AAP Publishes New Policies to Boost Child Immunization Rates" (2016). www.healthychildren.org.

2. De Vrese, M., et al. (2005). Probiotic bacteria stimulate virus-specific neutralizing antibodies following a booster polio vaccination. *Eur. J. Nutr., 44,* 406–413.
3. Soh, S. E., et al. (2010). Effect of probiotic supplementation in the first 6 months of life on specific antibody responses to infant hepatitis B vaccination. *Vaccine, 28,* 2577–2579.
4. Licciardi, P. V., et al. (2013). Maternal supplementation with LGG reduces vaccine-specific immune responses in infants at high-risk of developing allergic disease. *Front. Immunol., 4,* 381.
5. Kukkonen, K., Nieminen, T., Poussa, T., Savilahti, E., & Kuitunen, M. (2006). Effect of probiotics on vaccine antibody responses in infancy: A randomized placebo-controlled double-blind trial. *Pediatr. Allergy Immunol., 17,* 416–421.
6. Mao, X., et al. (2016). Dietary Lactobacillus rhamnosus GG supplementation improves the mucosal barrier function in the intestine of weaned piglets challenged by porcine rotavirus. *PloS One, 11,* e0146312.
7. Davidson, L. E., Fiorino, A.-M., Snydman, D. R., & Hibberd, P. L. (2011). Lactobacillus GG as an immune adjuvant for live-attenuated influenza vaccine in healthy adults: A randomized double-blind placebo-controlled trial. *Eur. J. Clin. Nutr., 65,* 501–507.

Chapter 12: Environment

1. Morass, B., Kiechl-Kohlendorfer, U., & Horak, E. (2008). The impact of early lifestyle factors on wheezing and asthma in Austrian preschool children. *Acta Paediatr., 97,* 337–341.
2. Stein, M. M., et al. (2016). Innate immunity and asthma risk in Amish and Hutterite farm children. *N. Engl. J. Med., 375,* 411–421.
3. Riedler, J., et al. (2001). Exposure to farming in early life and development of asthma and allergy: A cross-sectional survey. *Lancet Lond. Engl., 358,* 1129–1133; Fall, T., et al. (2015). Early exposure to dogs and farm animals and the risk of childhood asthma. *JAMA Pediatr., 169,* e153219; Von Mutius, E. (2007). Allergies, infections and the hygiene hypothesis: The epidemiological evidence. *Immunobiology, 212,* 433–439.
4. Stein, M. M., et al. (2016). Innate immunity and asthma risk in Amish and Hutterite farm children. *N. Engl. J. Med., 375,* 411–421.
5. Fall, T., et al. (2015). Early exposure to dogs and farm animals and the risk of childhood asthma. *JAMA Pediatr., 169,* e153219.
6. Fujimura, K. E., et al. (2014). House dust exposure mediates gut microbiome Lactobacillus enrichment and airway immune defense against allergens and virus infection. *Proc. Natl. Acad. Sci., 111,* 805–810.

7.   Fall, T., et al. (2015). Early exposure to dogs and farm animals and the risk of childhood asthma. *JAMA Pediatr., 169*, e153219.

8.   Song, S. J., et al. (2013). Cohabiting family members share microbiota with one another and with their dogs. *eLife, 2*, e00458.

9.   Lax, S., et al. (2014). Longitudinal analysis of microbial interaction between humans and the indoor environment. *Science, 345*, 1048–1052.

10.   Krezalek, M. A., DeFazio, J., Zaborina, O., Zaborin, A., & Alverdy, J. C. (2016). The shift of an intestinal "microbiome" to a "pathobiome" governs the course and outcome of sepsis following surgical injury. *Shock, 45*, 475–482.

11.   Lynch, S. J., Sears, M. R., & Hancox, R. J. (2016). Thumb-sucking, nail-biting, and atopic sensitization, asthma, and hay fever. *Pediatrics*. doi:10.1542/peds.2016-0443.

12.   Yee, A. L., & Gilbert, J. A. (2016). Microbiome. Is triclosan harming your microbiome? *Science, 353*, 348–349.

13.   Poole, et al. (2016) *mSphere, 1*, 3.

14.   Hospodsky, D., et al. (2014). Hand bacterial communities vary across two different human populations. *Microbiology, 160*, 1144–1152.

15.   Gibbons, S. M., et al. (2015). Ecological succession and viability of human-associated microbiota on restroom surfaces. *Appl. Environ. Microbiol., 81*, 765–773.

16.   Miranda, R. C., & Schaffner, D. W. (2016). Longer contact times increase cross-contamination of Enterobacter aerogenes from surfaces to food. *Appl. Environ. Microbiol., 82*, 6490–6496.

17.   Morass, B., Kiechl-Kohlendorfer, U., & Horak, E. (2008). The impact of early lifestyle factors on wheezing and asthma in Austrian preschool children. *Acta Paediatr., 97*, 337–341.

18.   Afshinnekoo, E., et al. (2015). Geospatial resolution of human and bacterial diversity with city-scale metagenomics. *Cell Syst., 1*, 97–97.e3.

19.   Hsu, T., et al. (2016). Urban transit system microbial communities differ by surface type and interaction with humans and the environment. *mSystems, 1*, e00018–16.

20.   Gonzalez, A., et al. (2016). Avoiding pandemic fears in the subway and conquering the platypus: Table 1. *mSystems, 1*, e00050–16.

21.   Hesselmar, B., Hicke-Roberts, A., & Wennergren, G. (2015). Allergy in children in hand versus machine dishwashing. *Pediatrics, 135*, e590–597.

22.   Kamimura, M., et al. (2016). The effects of daily bathing on symptoms of patients with bronchial asthma. *Asia Pac. Allergy, 6*, 112–119.

23.   Costello, E. K., Gordon, J. I., Secor, S. M., & Knight, R. (2010). Post-

prandial remodeling of the gut microbiota in Burmese pythons. *ISME J., 4,* 1375–1385.

24.   Thaiss, C. A., et al. (2014). Transkingdom control of microbiota diurnal oscillations promotes metabolic homeostasis. *Cell, 159,* 514–529.

25.   Leone, V., et al. (2015). Effects of diurnal variation of gut microbes and high-fat feeding on host circadian clock function and metabolism. *Cell Host Microbe, 17,* 681–689.

26.   Korves, T. M., et al. (2013). Bacterial communities in commercial aircraft high-efficiency particulate air (HEPA) filters assessed by PhyloChip analysis. *Indoor Air, 23,* 50–61.

27.   Kembel, S. W., et al. (2014). Architectural design drives the biogeography of indoor bacterial communities. *PLoS One, 9,* e87093.

Chapter 13: Conditions

1.   Yan, M., et al. (2013). Nasal microenvironments and interspecific interactions influence nasal microbiota complexity and S. aureus carriage. *Cell Host Microbe, 14,* 631–640.

2.   Zipperer, A., et al. (2016). Human commensals producing a novel antibiotic impair pathogen colonization. *Nature, 535,* 511–516.

3.   Fall, T., et al. (2015). Early exposure to dogs and farm animals and the risk of childhood asthma. *JAMA Pediatr., 169,* e153219.

4.   Fujimura, K. E., et al. (2014). House dust exposure mediates gut microbiome Lactobacillus enrichment and airway immune defense against allergens and virus infection. *Proc. Natl. Acad. Sci., 111,* 805–810.

5.   Stein, M. M., et al. (2016). Innate immunity and asthma risk in Amish and Hutterite farm children. *N. Engl. J. Med., 375,* 411–421.

6.   Arrieta, M.-C., et al. (2015). Early infancy microbial and metabolic alterations affect risk of childhood asthma. *Sci. Transl. Med., 7,* 307ra152.

7.   Fujimura, K. E., et al. (2016). Neonatal gut microbiota associates with childhood multisensitized atopy and T cell differentiation. *Nat. Med., 22,* 1187–1191.

8.   Hsiao, E. Y., et al. (2013). Microbiota modulate behavioral and physiological abnormalities associated with neurodevelopmental disorders. *Cell, 155,* 1451–1463.

9.   Kang, D.-W., et al. (2013). Reduced incidence of Prevotella and other fermenters in intestinal microflora of autistic children. *PLoS One, 8,* e68322.

10.   Teng, F., et al. (2015). Prediction of early childhood caries via spatial-temporal variations of oral microbiota. *Cell Host Microbe, 18,* 296–306.

11. Pozo-Rubio, T., et al. (2013). Influence of early environmental factors on lymphocyte subsets and gut microbiota in infants at risk of celiac disease; the PROFICEL study. *Nutr. Hosp., 28,* 464–473.

12. Davis-Richardson, A. G., et al. (2014). Bacteroides dorei dominates gut microbiome prior to autoimmunity in Finnish children at high risk for type 1 diabetes. *Front. Microbiol., 5,* 678.

Conclusion: A Few Words on Hype

1. Reber, S. O., et al. (2016). Immunization with a heat-killed preparation of the environmental bacterium *Mycobacterium vaccae* promotes stress resilience in mice. *Proc. Natl. Acad. Sci., 113,* E3130–E3139.

2. Sivan, A., et al. (2015). Commensal Bifidobacterium promotes antitumor immunity and facilitates anti-PD-L1 efficacy. *Science, 350,* 1084–1089.